An Introduction to the U.S. Health Care System

Third Edition

STEVEN JONAS is Professor of Preventive Medicine, School of Medicine, State University of New York at Stony Brook, where he has been a faculty member since 1971. Born and educated in New York City, he received his B.A. from Columbia College in 1958, his M.D. from the Harvard Medical School in 1962, and his M.P.H. from the Yale School of Medicine in 1967.

He is a Fellow of the American College of Preventive Medicine, the American Public Health Association, and the New York Academy of Medicine. He is an Associate Editor of *Preventive Medicine* and the *American Journal of Preventive Medicine* and Book Review Editor of the *American Journal*. He is a past-president of the Association of Teachers of Preventive Medicine and a past member of the New York State Board for Medicine.

Among his previous books are *Quality Control of Ambulatory Care* (New York: Springer Publishing Co., 1977), and *Medical Mystery: The Training of Doctors in the United States* (New York: W. W. Norton, 1978). He is founding editor, and editor and coauthor of the first three editions, of *Health Care Delivery in the United States,* also published by Springer. On health policy, Dr. Jonas has published over 100 professional articles and book reviews and has delivered over 50 papers at conferences and seminars. He has also published several books and numerous articles on sport, exercise, and weight loss.

An Introduction to the U.S. Health Care System

Third Edition

Steven Jonas, MD, MPH

1st and 2nd Editions
by **Milton Roemer,** *MD, MPH*

Springer Publishing Company

New York

To those whose pathways I've tried to follow: Dick Weinerman, Milt Roemer, Jeff Freymann, and Rosemary Stevens.

Springer Publishing Company, Inc.
536 Broadway
New York, NY 10012-3955

94 95 / 5

Jonas, Steven.
   An introduction to the U.S. health care system / Steven Jonas.—3rd ed.
      p. cm.
   Rev. ed. of: An introduction to the U.S. health care system / Milton I. Roemer.
   ISBN 0-8261-3984-1
   1. Medical care—United States. I. Roemer, Milton Irwin, 1916- Introduction to the U.S. health care system. II. Title. III. Title: Introduction to the US health care system.
RA395.A3J654 1991   91-15830
   362.1'0973—dc20   CIP

Printed in the United States of America

Contents

Contributor

Milton I. Roemer has been a Professor at the School of Public Health of the University of California, Los Angeles, since 1962. He taught previously at the Cornell University Institute of Hospital Administration (1957–61) and at Yale Medical School (1949–51). Dr. Roemer earned the M.D. degree in 1940 and also holds master's degrees in sociology and in public health.

Dr. Roemer has served at all levels of health administration—as a County Health Officer in West Virginia, a state and provincial health official in New Jersey and Saskatchewan, Canada, a commissioned officer of the U.S. Public Health Service in Washington, and a Section Chief of the World Health Organization headquarters in Geneva, Switzerland. In 1974 he was elected to the Institute of Medicine of the National Academy of Sciences.

As a consultant to international agencies, Dr. Roemer has studied health care organization in 61 countries on all the continents. He is the author of 32 books and over 400 articles on the social aspects of medicine. In 1977, he was the recipient of the American Public Health Association International Award for Excellence in Promoting and Protecting the Health of People. In 1983, the APHA awarded Dr. Roemer its highest honor, the Sedgwick Memorial Medal for Distinguished Service in Public Health.

Foreword to the Third Edition

This third edition of *An Introduction to the U.S. Health Care System*, like the system itself, shows further development. Even more than the first two editions, it portrays the "system as a whole," complicated but still described and analyzed as a total organism.

With the sophistication and clarity of Dr. Steven Jonas, this account manages to encompass all the diverse components of the American health system in a relatively short volume. It paints a picture with the necessary highlights and shadows, yet on a canvas within a relatively small frame. The different parts of the landscape blend gracefully together as in a painting of Rembrandt or Van Gogh.

Much writing on the American health system is out of balance. It focuses on some special aspect or views things under a special lens that distorts reality. This book, by contrast, is balanced and fair; it does not miss the forest for the trees. It sees the health system as a total living body that reflects the social, economic, and cultural circumstances around it, just as Darwin showed the adaptation of animal life to its environment.

In painting this picture, Dr. Jonas does not limit the colors to his preferences. On virtually every aspect, he presents the views of other scholars or leaders whose work has contributed to shaping the system. The extensive quotations are carefully selected, not to support the author's viewpoint but to record widely accepted judgments on various controversial issues (of which there are plenty).

Health systems, like scientific medicine or sociology, tend to breed a great deal of technical jargon. Old-timers often enjoy this because it makes them feel important by puzzling the newcomer. But this book carefully avoids such jargon, replacing it with down-to-earth language. If an acronym such as HMO (health maintenance organization) or DRG (diagnosis-related group) is used, the term that the letters stand for is always given. More important, the meaning of the term is explained so that one can understand why it was used in the first place.

The first edition of this book appeared in 1982, and ten years later we have the third edition. This simple fact shows how rapidly the U.S. health-care system is changing. Almost as we read about it the system is becoming increasingly organized and increasingly developed in a constant battle to respond to unmet human needs. The strategies used to fight that battle may not always be the most effective in your opinion or mine, but there is no question about a simple truth: If society's needs are not met, social problems are perceived. When these problems are clearly understood, they lead to change. This is certainly true about the U.S. system of health care. This small book can help everyone to understand that system—its characteristics, its problems, and possible improvements.

MILTON I. ROEMER, M.D., M.P.H.

Preface to the Third Edition

This is the third edition of *An Introduction to the U.S. Health Care System*. It is my privilege and honor to succeed Dr. Milton Roemer as the principal author of this book. In 1966, then a student at the Yale School of Public Health, I went to my first American Public Health Association annual meeting, that year in Los Angeles. My mentor, the late Dr. E. Richard Weinerman, had me in tow and introduced me to all the greats, the luminaries of the field that was then called Medical Care. None shone more brightly than Dr. Roemer. As I said in a letter to him after we came to final agreement on doing this book together, I feel like the kid who idolized the superstar baseball player and then grew up to play on the same team with him.

This edition is a substantial revision of Dr. Roemer's previous work. Except for Chapter 9, written entirely by him, I take full responsibility for the contents of the book. It does draw significantly on previously published work of myself and of Dr. Roemer. The material from the second edition is used with the kind permission of Dr. Roemer and with my thanks to him. Earlier versions of certain portions of the text written by me for this book appeared in parts that I wrote of the second, third, and to a very limited extent fourth editions of *Health Care Delivery in the United States*.* That text is used with the permission of the publisher and copyright holder, the Springer Publishing Co.

This book describes the U.S. health-care delivery system in broad outline. It focuses on principles, basic structures, and important unsolved problems. It is not concerned with the specifics of current

---

Health Care Delivery in the United States provides in-depth description and analysis of the subject, in contrast with the introductory approach that this book takes. I edited the second and third editions of *HCDUS*, published in 1981 and 1986, respectively. The current fourth edition is edited by my friend and colleague Anthony Kovner, Ph.D. It was published by the Springer Publishing Co. in 1990.

legislative proposals and programs and how they are or are not being implemented. It takes a primarily qualitative rather than quantitative approach. Thus, while it uses some numbers, it uses them lightly. It is referenced, but it does not have a profusion of citations. For a more comprehensive approach, more quantitative information, and many more references, readers are referred to the fourth edition of *Health Care Delivery in the United States.*

As have the first two editions, this book is intended for use in undergraduate courses on the U.S. health-care delivery system and graduate survey courses, for teaching the subject to medical students, (who usually do not cover it in any depth if they cover it at all), and for the practicing health professional who simply wants an overview of the system.

Although *An Introduction* is not a policy book, Dr. Roemer and I have written a great deal on policy. Thus this book has a political and philosophical point of view. Although it always attempts to be objective, it is not neutral. Its primary social value is that the principal purpose of the U.S. health-care delivery system is to meet and serve the health-care needs of the American people.

At various points in the course of the book, proposals for U.S. health-care policy and program changes are described. Very occasionally, some are recommended. I hope that after assimilating the factual material presented, you will be able to come to your own conclusions about what is to be done. I am certain that if nothing else, you will agree with the majority of the American people that something must be done to reform both the structure and the functions of the system.

Chapter 1 provides an overview of the system. Chapters 2 and 3 cover its primary outpatient and inpatient institutions and institutional forms. Chapter 4 presents the people who provide the care. Chapter 5 covers governmental roles and functions; 6, the principles of health planning. Financing is reviewed in Chapter 7, and the history of and prospects for national health insurance in the United States are covered in Chapter 8. Dr. Roemer puts the U.S. system in the world context in Chapter 9.

I am pleased to acknowledge the support of my department chairman, Dr. Andre Varma, for this project. My father, Professor Harold J. Jonas, has once again provided expert editing services. I thank Mrs. Betsy Pollert for her dedicated effort in word processing, and my secretary, Mrs. Lola Michelini, for her help in many different ways. I thank Dr. Gail Kuhn Weisman for her assistance in preparing the section on nursing personnel.

At Springer, I thank my hardworking editor, Ms. Kathleen O'Malley; Ms. Barbara Watkins, who was instrumental in arranging for the passage of the torch from Dr. Roemer to me; and last, but never least, the woman without whom none of this work would ever have seen the light of day, Dr. Ursula Springer.

STEVEN JONAS, M.D., M.P.H.

Abbreviations

AALL	—	American Association for Labor Legislation
AAMC	—	Association of American Medical Colleges
ADAMHA	—	Alcohol, Drug Abuse, and Mental Health Administration
AFDC	—	Aid to Families with Dependent Children
AHA	—	American Hospital Association
ALOS	—	Average Length of Stay
AMA	—	American Medical Association
ANA	—	American Nurses' Association
ASTHO	—	Association of State and Territorial Health Officials
CCMC	—	Committee on the Costs of Medical Care
CDC	—	Center for Disease Control
CHAMPUS	—	Civilian Health and Medical Program of the Uniformed Services
CHC	—	Community Health Center
CHSS	—	Cooperative Health Statistics System
CME	—	Continuing Medical Education
DHEW	—	Department of Health, Education and Welfare
DHHS	—	Department of Health and Human Services
D.O.	—	Doctor of Osteopathy
DOD	—	Department of Defense
DRG	—	Diagnosis Related Group
DVA	—	Department of Veterans Affairs
EMS	—	Emergency Medical Service (or System)
EMT	—	Emergency Medical Technician
ER	—	Emergency Room
FDA	—	Food and Drug Administration
FSMB	—	Federation of State Medical Boards
GAC	—	General Accounting Office
GHI	—	Group Health Insurance
GMENAC	—	Graduate Medical Education National Advisory Committee
GNP	—	Gross National Product
GPEP	—	General Professional Education of the Physician Panel
HANES	—	Health and Nutrition Examination Survey

HCFA	— Health Care Financing Administration
HHS	— Health and Human Services
HIAA	— Health Insurance Association of America
HIP	— Health Insurance Plan
HMO	— Health Maintenance Organization
HRA	— Health Resources Administration; Health Risk Appraisal
HRSA	— Health Resources and Services Administration
IPA	— Individual or Independent Practice Association
JCAH	— Joint Commission on Accreditation of Hospitals
LCME	— Liaison Committee on Medical Education
LHD	— Local Health Department
LPN	— Licensed Pratical Nurse
MCH	— Maternal and Child Health
MMWR	— *Morbidity and Mortality Weekly Report*
MVSR	— *Monthly Vital Statistics Report*
NCHS	— National Center for Health Statistics
NHC	— Neighborhood Health Center
NHI	— National Health Insurance
NHS	— National Health Survey or Service (check the context)
NIH	— National Institutes of Health
NIMH	— National Institute of Mental Health
NLN	— National League for Nursing
NP	— Nurse Practitioner
OEO	— Office of Economic Opportunity
OMB	— Office of Management and Budget
PA	— Physicians' Assistant (or Associate)
PHCS	— Personal Health Care System
PHS	— Public Health Service
PPGP	— Prepaid Group Practice
PPO	— Preferred Provider Organization
RN	— Registered Nurse
SHA	— State Health Agency
USDA	— United States Department of Agriculture
USDHEW	— United States Department of Health, Education and Welfare
USDHHS	— United States Department of Health and Human Services
USGPO	— United States Government Printing Office
USPHS	— United States Public Health Service
VA	— Veterans Administration
WHO	— World Health Organization

Chapter **1**

The U.S. Health Care Delivery System: An Overview

MAJOR DEFINING CHARACTERISTICS

Several major characteristics of the system of health care in the United States distinguish it from that of most of the world's 160 or so other nations. First, the United States is an affluent industrialized country, and it has chosen to spend much money on health services. In fact it spends a higher proportion of its Gross National Product— 11.1 percent in 1988 (Office of National Cost Estimates)—than any other country in the world. Second, since the United States is a federated nation, the system's governance is decentralized to many states, counties, and communities. Third, this nation has a freer market economy than most other countries. Thus, in the operations of most of the system's components, permissive laissez-faire concepts have been the norm, at least until very recently.

There are, of course, other affluent and industrialized nations, other federated republics, and other relatively laissez-faire economies. The degree to which these attributes have influenced the U.S. health-care system, however, is significant. The system is pluralistic and complex. It delivers a product which varies widely in quantity and quality by region and social class of its recipients.

The origins of the federated political structure can be traced to the American Revolution against the British monarchy. The founders of the Republic were determined to avoid creating a central government that was too strong. Thus governmental sovereignty is split between the central government and the states (see Chapter 5). Within the central government there are "checks and balances" between

1

the executive, legislative, and judicial branches which restrain governmental actions of all types.

The free-market economy was emerging in Europe in the early nineteenth century just when the New World was beginning to develop. Inevitably these dynamic economic processes influenced the American health-care system. National and health professional leaders have generally been dedicated to free-market principles. Yet in spite of that, many interventions in the operation of the market for health services have become necessary. The expectations of people for recovery from disease and the maintenance of good health have risen. As this has occurred, more initiatives to change the contours of the system's parts have become necessary. Social actions have been taken to increase the quantity and quality of resources produced, to plan for and change system management, to alter the overall system structure, to strengthen mechanisms of financial support, and to rationalize and improve the delivery of services.

American medical practice is organized primarily on the private entrepreneurial model. Although with the advent of health maintenance organizations the pattern is changing (see Chapter 2), medical care is provided primarily on the basis of a private, direct contract between physician and patient. It is usually unwritten, even when the source of payment is not the patient. Since medical care—that is, the treatment of sick persons by physicians—is the focus of the U.S. health-care system and primarily private, the organizational framework of the health-care system is rudimentary compared to that found in other countries. But before reviewing some of the details of the system, let us consider some of the characteristics of the population it serves.

THE HEALTH STATUS OF THE U.S. POPULATION*

In 1988 the U.S. population was about 246 million (*Stat.*, Table 2). The population is aging; the proportion of persons 65 and over is over 12 percent (*Stat.*, Table 13). Many ethnic and national groups are represented. There is a broad range of social classes, and large income differentials exist. There are also great inequities in the amount

---

*Unless otherwise referenced, the data presented in the balance of this chapter come from the *Statistical Abstract of the United States*, 110th ed. (Washington, DC: U.S. Bureau of the Census, 1990), cited in the text as *Stat.*, and *Health United States, 1989*, (Hyattsville, MD: U.S. Department of Health and Human Services [USDHHS], Pub. No. [PHS] 90–1232, March, 1990), cited in the text as *Health*.

and quality of health care received and in health status. Much of the excellent health service of which the nation is capable is not accessible to everyone. Proportionately, there are more nonwhite persons in the lower class and income groups than in the general population. Unemployment, or the threat of it, substandard housing, and dysnutrition are major socioeconomic problems in rural and urban areas.

In 1988 overall life expectancy for U.S. residents was 74.9 years at birth (*Stat.*, Table 103). For men it was 71.4 years; for women, 78.3 years. There was a marked difference in life expectancy at birth by race: 75.5 for whites, 71.5 for blacks. (Ominously, in 1989, for the first time in many years. U.S. life expectancy declined [Hilts; MVSR]. And the black-white gap widened. At that time it was of course too early to know whether this was a one-time artifact or an event of historical significance.) The black-white difference in life expectancy is thought in part to reflect differences in the standard of living as well as access to health services (Schwartz et al.).

In 1988 the U.S. infant mortality rate was 9.9 per 1,000 live births (*Stat.*, Table 80). While this is low, it is slightly higher than that of some 14 other countries, mainly in Western Europe, but including Australia, Canada, and Japan (*Stat.*, Table 1440). It is perhaps significant that in 1987, other than Switzerland, Japan, and Germany, these countries had a lower per capita gross national product than the United States. However, they all have systems of national health care which make services accessible to virtually everyone at little or no cost at the time of service. The white-black infant mortality rate difference in the United States is striking. In 1987, it was 8.6 for whites, 15.4 for blacks (*Stat.*, Table 110). However, the black infant mortality rate has been double that for whites since 1915 when the rate was first recorded, and it was 99.9 overall (Grove & Hetzel).

In 1988 the crude death rate was under 9 per 1,000 population—9.4 for males, 8.3 for females (*Stat.*, Table 107). Again, there was a major differential by ethnic group. The *crude* death rate was higher for whites, 9.1, than it was for blacks, 8.5. But the *age-adjusted* death rates (which statistically account for the fact that black life expectancy is shorter) were 5.1 for whites, 7.1 for blacks. The major causes of death in the general population are heart disease, cancer, stroke, personal injury, and chronic obstructive lung disease and pneumonia (*Stat.*, Table 115). The major causes of morbidity (sickness) are upper respiratory infections, influenza, injuries, heart conditions, hypertension, arthritis, impairments of the lower limbs, impairments of the back and spine, asthma and hay fever, and mild emotional disorders (Adams & Hardy, Tables 1–10).

There is no consistent association between family income and the number of acute conditions per 100 persons per year. However, there is an inverse correlation between family income and the number of days of restricted activity associated with acute conditions (Adams & Hardy, Tables 4, 19). It is interesting to note that blacks report both fewer acute conditions and fewer days of restricted activity than do whites (Adams & Hardy, Tables 3, 18). There are no statistically significant differences by either ethnicity or income in the proportion of persons with acute illnesses receiving medical attention (Adams & Hardy, Tables 13, 14).

THE ELEMENTS OF THE SYSTEM

Any health-care delivery system has five major components: health-care institutions, personnel who work in them, firms producing "health commodities" such as pharmaceutical drugs and hospital equipment, institutions that produce biomedical knowledge and health personnel, and the financing mechanism. In addition, there is an organizational structure standing at the system's center, like the trunk of a tree. (In the United States there is not one central trunk but multiple ones. Think banyan tree, not oak.) It is this structure which enables the components to interact and function to produce health services for the people.

A major element of the organizational structure is the system of management. Among the industrialized countries of the world, that system is unique. There is no national Ministry of Health playing a central role in the financing and operation of health services. In other countries, even if the ministry does not operate the system directly, it at least creates and supervises the structure within which it functions. There is no equivalent in the United States. There is of course a system; there are loci of power and control, but they are sometimes difficult to recognize and describe.

HEALTH SERVICES COMPONENTS

In this section we briefly consider each of the five major components of the health care delivery system: institutions, manpower, commodities, knowledge and personnel production, and financing. The principal ones are treated in separate chapters.

Health-Care Institutions

Various types of institutions provide health-care services. The most frequently used type of care is "ambulatory," provided to patients other than those in institutional beds. About 60 percent of ambulatory care is delivered in private doctors' offices; other sites include hospital ambulatory services (about 13%), by telephone (about 14%), the home (about 1.5%), and "other," (group practices, health maintenance organization, neighborhood health centers, and local health department health centers), about 13 percent (*Health,* Table 64). (For more detail, see Chapter 2).

Of the institutions housing and caring for patients in bed, acute-care hospitals are the most numerous. In 1989, there were about 5,800, with about 1.04 million beds (AHA, Table 1). Hospitals are categorized in a variety of ways: ownership, size, function, and average length of stay. There are three principal types of ownership: government (federal, state, and local); private, not-for-profit (voluntary); and private, for-profit (proprietary). There are four functional categories for hospitals in the United States: general, tuberculosis, mental, and other special. The American Hospital Association also defines the "community hospital": a nonfederal, short-term general or other special hospital. It is the predominant type in the United States. Hospitals are covered in Chapter 3. Nursing homes and other nonmental-condition long-term institutions, of which there were about 16,000 in 1986, plus other long-term services, are briefly described in Chapter 3.

Health Manpower

In 1988, about 8.8 million people worked in the health-care system (*Health,* Table 83). The largest groups are the nurses, clerical staff, hospital manual workers, physicians, dentists, pharmacists, and technicians. The physicians, of whom there were more than 560,000 active in 1987, are the most powerful group. Health manpower is covered in Chapter 4.

Health Commodities

A wide variety of commodities are used in the health-care system. Many kinds of equipment and supplies for the diagnosis and treatment of disease are produced by the hospital and medical-supply manufacturers. These items range from gauze pads, sterile needles, laboratory chemicals, and anesthetic gases, to diagnostic imaging and laboratory equipment, surgical instruments, orthopedic appliances, eyeglasses, hearing aids, dental prostheses, and hospital furniture. The other major category of health commodity is pharmaceutical drugs. (For a brief essay on the pharmaceutical industry, please see Addendum I of Chapter 5, Government.)

Health Personnel and Knowledge Reproduction

Every health-care system depends on knowledge about health and disease, and the application of that knowledge to prevention and treatment through various technologies. A vast store of knowledge has been gathered from the observations and experience of past centuries, but in the modern world new knowledge is constantly being acquired by scientific research. Knowledge must be activated by the education and training of people to use it. Health-sciences education plays a critical role in forming the health-care system (medical education is touched upon in Chapter 4, Health Manpower.)

Health Economics and Financing

In 1988 the United States spent about $540 billion on health services, more than 11 percent of its gross national product (GNP) (Office of National Cost Estimates, 1–5). Since the passage in 1965 of Medicare legislation (providing for payment for certain health-care services to person 65 and older under Social Security), inflation in health-care costs has consistently outstripped general inflation (Office of National Cost Estimates, Figure 4).

Ultimately, all money paid for health services comes from the people. There are three major means by which money is transferred from them to the providers of health services: (1) government (in 1988 about 42% of total expenditures); (2) insurance companies (about 32% of the total); and (3) direct payment (about 26% of the total) (Office of National Cost Estimates, Figure 2). Government expenditures are for services that it operates directly and services patients receive from independent providers. In this case government is a "third-party" payor (that is, neither the provider nor the patient but simply the payor). The two major factors in the private insurance sector are Blue Cross/Blue Shield (not-for-profit) and commercial (for-profit) companies.

The major recipients of funds are hospitals (39%), physicians (19%), nursing homes (8%), other personal health care (22%), and other spending (12%) (Office of National Cost Estimates, Figure 2).

The majority of health-care personnel are paid on salary; the private practitioners are usually paid on a fee-for-service basis. Institutions for the most part operate on a global budget or on a cost-reimbursement basis. I cover financing mechanisms in more detail in Chapter 8.

ORGANIZATIONAL STRUCTURE
Management of the Resources

If institutions, personnel, and financing are to be brought together to provide health care, they must be managed. System management in this context includes four major activities: planning, administration, regulation, and evaluation. Each of these activities is closely related to the others. It should be noted that these terms are not used consistently throughout all parts of the health-care system. A given action may be termed *deliberate planning* in one part, *normal administration* in a second, and *official regulation* in a third.

Planning

Planning is any deliberate governmental or nongovernmental action for the allocation of resources in some systematic way (outside the mechanisms of the free market) to accomplish stated goals and objectives. In this sense, health planning in the United States and elsewhere can be said to have occurred with the establishment of the first hospital or the organization of the first department of public health. As customarily used, however, *health planning* refers to the actions of an agency which functions over and above the health resources and health organizations themselves, exerting an influence on their courses of action. In this sense, health planning in the United States has been very weak indeed. It has been largely confined to hospital construction, and the decisions have been made by agencies that are both local and nongovernmental.

Since the midsixties when the national hospital construction program, called Hill-Burton after its two principal congressional sponsors, came to an end, government has had two primary roles. One has been to issue "guidelines" (rather than regulations or official standards). The other has been to say "No, you cannot do that" rather than "Yes, to meet these identified needs, you should do this, and here's some money to help."

Draft federal guidelines covering the types and characteristics of health services, goals to be achieved through the health-planning process, were developed for the first time under the Carter administration and released in 1979 (USDHEW, 1979). Also established were specific health-status goals to be achieved by the system. The latter were retained by the Reagan administration in another form; the former were discarded. (For a discussion of the principles of health planning, see Chapter 6.)

Regulation

Somewhat paradoxically, in the United States health-care regulation is highly developed. To some extent because of the highly decentralized administrative structure, many problems and abuses have developed. In response, regulations have been imposed to prevent further abuses. It should be understood that government regulation is a reactive not a proactive process. It usually comes into effect only after some player undertakes an activity which either upsets a relatively level economic playing field or undertakes an activity which undermines the health, safety, or comfort of some significant group of people in the society.

Evaluation

Evaluation has also become highly developed in the U.S. health-care system for reasons similar to the development of the regulatory system. So much freedom has characterized the delivery of health services, and their costs have risen so rapidly, that many people were bound to raise questions about the quality and value of those services. As the role of government and large groups in the financing of health services decreased and the role of the individual declined, the questions became more insistent. As a response, various methods of evaluation have been developed in the U.S. health services system (see chapter 14, "The Quality of Care," by Beth C. Weitzman, in the fourth edition of *Health Care Delivery in the United States*).

Administration

The administration of health services is a complex matter, itself the subject of many lengthy books. As an example of its complexity, let us briefly consider here the administration of ambulatory (outpatient) services found in a typical teaching (medical school-affiliated) hospital with an emergency unit and clinics. There are ordinarily three vertical organizational lines: medical staff; nursing staff; and business administration, housekeeping, dietary, maintenance and other support services. Sometimes these vertical lines meet in the director's office; sometimes they never meet; occasionally they are well integrated.

This structure is reflected in the organization of ambulatory services. Generally, each medical department is responsible for physician services in its own clinics. The pattern may extend to the emergency unit, or it may be the primary responsibility of one department, say, surgery. Alternatively, physician staffing in the emergency unit may be entirely the responsibility of an emergency department. This department may stand on its own, be part of a department of ambulatory services or community medicine, or be attached to the office of the hospital's director. In teaching hospitals, departments of ambulatory services, when they exist, may exert some control over emergency physicians, but only rarely do they have any true control over clinic physician staffing.

The nursing department generally controls the nursing services for both clinics and emergency units, sometimes appointing an associate or assistant director of nursing for ambulatory care. Likewise, the hospital's administration runs the clerical and other support services, often through an associate or assistant administrator or director. This tripartite approach works well as long as there is no special interest in establishing one coordinated *program* in ambulatory care.

This situation reflects a more general administrative problem with which hospitals around the country are wrestling. Its resolution will require major changes in the way hospitals are structured. Those structural changes will in turn require major changes in the way people think and feel. With a few exceptions, hospitals are not used to mounting coordinated *programs* but to delivering *services*, each component putting in its piece more or less as it sees fit. Most importantly, medical staff is used to functioning independently, not as part of a hospital team. Many of the present contradictions evident in the role and work of service, teaching, and research in hospitals will have to be resolved before these administrative problems can be solved. (See Chapters 4, Hospitals, and 6, Planning.)

HEALTH PROGRAMS

The output of any health-care delivery system is often described in terms of its major "health programs." The forms and proportionate role of each program differ among national systems. In the United

States as in most countries there are five major types of health program, those of the principal governmental health authority, other agencies of government with health functions, voluntary health agencies, commercial enterprises with health functions, and the private health-care sector. It is within the health programs that the five components—facilities, personnel, commodities, knowledge, and money—interact to produce health services.

Government in Health Services

Although the government by itself operates no program of the health-care system in its entirety, it is closely involved in one way or another in all of them by collecting and disseminating information, educating and training personnel directly and providing financial support; operating health-care institutions; providing other direct health services; participating in financing, supporting, and carrying out research, planning, evaluating, and regulating.

When the need to protect people from hazards of the environment and epidemic diseases was recognized, public health agencies were developed. Social insurance began as a movement to protect the economic position of low-paid workers, who could be ruined by the costs of sickness—both lost earnings and the costs of medical care. Almost everywhere, therefore, the locus of social insurance in the structure of government has been different from that of public health.

The principal health agency of the U.S. federal government is the Department of Health and Human Services, headed by a cabinet-level secretary. It is responsible for the federal Social Security program, the federal role in the state-run public assistance programs, and the main federal programs in health services, research, regulation, and financing. Many of the department's responsibilities are met by allocation of money and delegation of authority to many other public and private entities throughout the nation. Because this country is a federation of states, the Constitution grants the states a great deal of autonomy and responsibility in all social affairs, including health.

The first U.S. national social insurance program to finance medical care, Medicare, was established in 1965. Originally, its operation was placed in the Social Security Administration (SSA), not the Public Health Service (PHS). Even when administration of the Medicare program was later withdrawn from the Social Security Administration, it was not placed in an agency concerned strictly with health but in another arm of the Department of Health and Human Services, the Health Care Financing Administration (HCFA). HCFA also runs

Medicaid, the state-federal program that provides some financing for some health services for some of the nation's poor.

In each of the 50 states there is a major health agency. In some states, as at the federal level, it is combined with authorities for social welfare or other functions. The administrative configuration and scope of functions of the state health agencies are highly variable. The heads of these agencies are ordinarily appointed by the governor. They are responsible entirely to the governor and not to the U.S. Department of Health and Human Services. Only insofar as certain standards must be met as a condition for receipt of certain federal monies must the state accept national direction. (Of course, under the federal-supremacy doctrine, the states may not undertake any actions that are contrary to the provisions of the Constitution.)

Similarly, below the level of state government, there are units of local government, counties, cities, and occasionally special districts that also have a major health agency. Most of these have great autonomy, although on certain health matters the local health department may carry out functions delegated by the state agency. For a closer look at government activities in health-care delivery see Chapters 5 and 7.

Voluntary Agencies

In all countries there are nongovernmental agencies that play a role in health-care systems. Commonly known as voluntary agencies (e.g., American Heart Association, American Cancer Society, Visiting Nurse Association), they have a wide variety of functions: to perform a service not rendered by other agencies, to pursue a certain research or service objective with special vigor and dedication, to advance or protect the interests of a certain population group, and sometimes to carry out certain tasks at the behest of official bodies. Like any corporation, to stay in business they must take in more money than they spend. In the "voluntary" agency, however, the excess of income over expenses does not accrue to any individual but supports the expansion of the agency's work. These corporation are thus termed *not-for-profit* or *nonprofit*.

In the United States there are hundreds of agencies that raise funds and carry out programs for fighting certain diseases (cancer, tuberculosis, mental illness); focusing on the health of certain population groups (children, Native Americans, veterans); providing certain types of health services (visiting-nurse care, hospitalization, rehabilitation). The voluntary agency may be devoted exclusively to health purposes, or health services may be incidental to certain larger purposes such as those of church groups or religious missions (domestic or foreign).

A subset of the voluntary health agency is the health professional organization; for example, the American Medical Association, the American Nurses Association, the American College of Preventive Medicine, the Academy for Health Services Marketing. They are financed by membership dues, journal subscriptions, and advertising fees, and on occasion research grants and contracts. They are primarily concerned with advancing the perceived professional and economic interests of their members through public education, continuing professional education, litigation, legislative and political action, and, on occasion, trade-unionlike activity. They may also focus on advancing scientific knowledge and understanding, setting and maintaining professional standards, and educating the public about health and disease.

For-Profit Enterprises with Health Functions

There are two classes of for-profit enterprises which provide health services: corporations which deliver health services to their employees and commercial entities which provide health services to the public.

Employee Health

In the United States, in-plant employee health services are generally of circumscribed scope, except in large establishments (more than 500 workers). In smaller factories, services are usually limited to first aid by an industrial nurse or perhaps only a medicine chest for self-use. Large plants or mines may maintain a staff of physicians and nurses who perform periodic and preplacement examinations; treat any intercurrent illness, whether or not job-connected; and promote education for healthful living. Enterprises in isolated locations, such as railroad junctions or lumber mills, may operate comprehensive medical-care programs. Industrial firms are obligated by law to protect workers from accidents and occupational diseases, although enforcement is often weak. (See Chapter 2, under "Industrial Health Service Units.")

For-Profit Health Service Enterprises

These play a significant role in the U.S. health-care system. There are four groups. (1) those engaged in "commodities production," mentioned above; (2) the private health and hospital insurance companies (see Chapter 8) and companies providing professional liability (malpractice) insurance protection; (3) the for-profit general hospitals (of which an increasing proportion is coming under for-profit control, about 14% of the general beds in 1988 [AHA, Table 1]; (4) nursing homes for the aged and chronically ill, long predominately proprietary, with 80 percent of their beds in units operated for profit.

Private Professional Practice

The U.S. health-care system is dominated by private professional practice. As of the 1990s, though system trends have been changing many of these relationships, office and in-hospital medical care (both general and specialized), dental care, chiropractic, pharmacy, optical, medical and nonmedical psychotherapeutic, speech and audiology services, fitting prosthetic appliances, and others are furnished primarily by private practitioners.

It is especially noteworthy that even when the financial support for health services has been collectivized as in the various public or voluntary health insurance programs or in the tax-supported Medicaid program for the poor, the provision of services remains substantially in the private market. For care in the doctor's private office, this is quite obvious, but even in a hospitalized case, the service is rendered to a private patient, and a responsible third-party payor pays a private fee. (For a further discussion of private medical practice, see Chapter 4).

DELIVERY OF HEALTH SERVICES

The several components of the health-care system, operating within the health-service programs, work together to produce health services for individuals and population groups. Health services are usually delivered by individual providers to individual patients. To distinguish the personal from the other parts of the system, this is customarily called "delivery of health services." These services are usually further categorized as primary, secondary, or tertiary.

Primary Care

In functional terms, primary care is that care which most people need most of the time for most of their health concerns. Primary health services include a wide range of personal preventive and treatment measure, in the industrialized countries usually provided by a physician.* Common forms of personal preventive measures are immunization, surveillance of expectant mothers and babies, and adult examination for detection of chronic diseases. Primary-care treatment covers most health services given to patients who are not in institutional beds, although there is some overlap in both directions. Primary care is discussed in more detail in Chapter 2.

Secondary and Tertiary Care

In the United States secondary and tertiary health-care services are highly developed. Until the past 25 years or so, any community or group that could raise the money to build a hospital and furnish the facility with whatever sophisticated diagnostic or treatment equipment it could afford was free to do so. The same freedom applied to physicians, who could specialize in whichever field they could find postgraduate training in. Thus, more than 85 percent of physicians became specialists.

Tertiary care, at the other end of the spectrum, consists of highly specialized diagnostic, therapeutic, and rehabilitative services requiring staff and equipment "that transcend the capabilities of the average community hospital" (Rogatz, 47). Such care, available largely at major medical centers, includes transplant surgery and other technologically complex procedures recently emerged from experimental status.

Secondary care, the most difficult level to define, includes services available at community hospitals or in private offices. Ideally they are arranged through referral or consultation after a preliminary evaluation by a primary-care practitioner. Secondary services include most surgery and the services of such specialists as radiologists, cardiologists, and endocrinologists.

Care of Special Populations and Disorders

In all health-care systems, there are special programs providing primary, secondary, and tertiary care for the care of certain population groups defined by age, sex, or occupation, and for the control of

---

*A *personal* health service is one given directly to an individual; e.g., treatment for an upper respiratory infection, the setting and casting of a fractured ankle. The recipient is almost invariably aware the she is receiving the service. The other class is community health service. This is provided for a group of people simultaneously. They may be aware that they are receiving it (e.g., public health education on smoking cessation) but are often unaware of that fact (e.g., the provision of a pure water supply and sanitary sewage disposal).

specific health disorders. In the United States private buying and selling of health service is the norm. In this light it is noteworthy that a number of special programs are provided by government. Among the categories of persons covered are military personnel and dependents, military service veterans, and Native Americans. These programs are covered briefly in Chapter 5.

Other populations for which special programs of health care have been created include railroad workers, migrant farm workers, certain industrial workers, schoolchildren, college and university students. Many of these programs are provided primarily by salaried personnel working in organized frameworks.

Mental illness is the most important health disorder for which special subsystems of health-care delivery are organized in the United States. In private practice, psychiatrists, clinical psychologists, and other therapists provide a great deal of ambulatory psychotherapy. Low-income patients receive such care if it is available from several thousand public or voluntary mental health clinics. Hospitalization for mental illness takes place primarily in special mental hospitals financed and operated by state governments (although community hospitals equipped to do so increasingly have been admitting short-term patients with psychiatric diagnoses). Tuberculosis, before its steep decline in incidence and prevalence, also warranted a special network of clinics and hospitals (sanitoriums) for its detection and care.

PROBLEMS IN HEALTH CARE DELIVERY IN THE UNITED STATES

For all of its resources, personnel, facilities, skills, knowledge, money, and ability to do wondrous things to and with the human body, U.S. health care is plagued with problems. Some observers call the situation a crisis. Sudden worsening is part of the definition of *crisis*, however, and the problems have been with us for a very long time. The health-care system is not in crisis. It has serious problems of long standing, some seemingly intractable.

It is fascinating that these problems are not those of a technical and/or scientific inability to deal with diseases or other health deficits. (There are a few exceptions to this rule, such as AIDS. But even in this case only *some* of the difficulties in controlling its spread are traceable to lack of knowledge or tools. For example, AIDS transmission among intravenous recreational mood-altering drug users could be cut sharply if (1) the drugs of choice were obtainable legally or (2) a comprehensive national clean-needle-exchange program was instituted. The choice not to do either is made on political, not medical or epidemiological grounds.) Nor is the problem one of lack of money, as it is in so many other countries.

In the U.S., the principal problems are that:

- We are spending too *much*, not too little.
- The rise in costs has been uncontrollable by any interventions tried to date.
- The distribution of health services is highly variable throughout the population.
- Much that could be done to prevent disease and promote health using available knowledge and techniques is not done.
- Many health-care needs are undermet (e.g., not enough home health care for the inform elderly), while others are overmet (e.g., too many hospital beds).

In short, the problems are not those of lack of resources but their misuse and misallocation. Neither providing more money nor artificially capping the amount of money spent is the solution. Rather, the *causes* of the misuse and misallocation must be identified and dealt with (see Chapters 7 and 8).

As far back as 1932, the findings of the first comprehensive study of health-care delivery in the United States were summarized in these terms (Committee on Costs of Medical Care, 2):

> The problem of providing satisfactory medical service to all the people of the United States at costs which they can meet is a pressing one. At the present time, many persons do not receive service which is adequate either in quantity or quality, and the costs of service are inequably distributed. The result is a tremendous amount of preventable physical pain and mental anguish, needless deaths, economic inefficiency, and social waste. Furthermore, these conditions are, as the following pages will show, largely unnecessary. The United States has the economic resources, the organizing ability, and the technical experience to solve this problem.

The committee, chaired by Ray Lyman Wilbur, a past president of the American Medical Association, had been created in 1927 to look into problems of health-delivery. Strikingly, some would say unfortunately, the statement is entirely applicable 60 years later.

In the 1960s and 1970s, observers of the U.S. health-care system of differing political persuasions often spoke of "crisis." Indeed there has been a long line of critical reports and studies going back many years. (For an introductory bibliography of such reports, see Appendix I.) For example, in 1968, an article, "Crisis in American Medicine," in the British journal *The Lancet* began (Battistella & Southby, 581):

In terms of gross national product the U.S.A. spends more on health than does any other country. But costs are rising at such a rate that more and more people will find it difficult to get complete health care. This particularly applies to the poor, the old, the Negroes, and other disadvantaged groups. Doctors and hospital beds are distributed most unevenly both in broad geographic regions and between States. There are indications, too, that the quality of care has been inferior, especially in terms of antenatal and infant mortality. The whole organization of medical care in the U.S.A. has failed to respond to changing disease patterns, the move from country to cities, industrialization, and the increasing proportion of old people in the population.

In 1970, the editors of *Fortune* wrote (9):

American medicine, the pride of the nation for many years, stands now on the brink of chaos. To be sure, our medical practitioners have their great moments of drama and triumph. But much of the U.S. medical care, particularly the everyday business of preventing and treating routine illnesses, is inferior in quality, wastefully dispensed, and inequitably financed. Medical manpower and facilities are so maldistributed that large segments of the population, especially the urban poor and those in rural areas, get virtually no care at all even though their illnesses are most numerous and, in a medical sense, often easy to cure.

In a similar vein, Senator Edward M. Kennedy, speaking to an audience of doctors in New York City in 1971, said (Klaw, xi):

America is beginning to realize that we have a health care crisis on our hands, and that the magnitude of the crisis is enormous. . . . I challenge even the most reactionary pillars of organized medicine, even the most affluent physicians in the most affluent suburbs of this rich city, to deny that a crisis exists, or that it exists for all Americans—not just the poor, not just the black, but each and every one of us.

In 1973, the Research and Policy Committee of the Committee for Economic Development, the board of which is composed of representatives of many of the leading American corporations and banks, came to the following conclusions concerning the present system (p. 17):

First, faulty allocation of resources is a major cause of inadequacies and inequalities in U.S. health services that result today in poor or substandard care for large segments of the population. Second, the task of assuring all people the ability to cope financially with the costs of health care has been made realizable by the substantial base of coverage now provided by both private and public insurance plans. Third, unless step-by-step alterations are made in the means of delivering services and paying providers, closing the gaps in financing would overburden an inadequate system and offer little prospect of materially improving the quality and quantity of medical services of the health of the American people.

In 1979, Congressman Ronald Dellums introduced a bill to create the National Health Service with a statement that said, in part (Dellums):

We have in this country today a health delivery system where the quality of health care received is determined by race, language, national origin, or income level. Health is viewed as a commodity to be bought and sold in the marketplace, it is not viewed as a right of the people; a service to be provided by the Government. However, financing is not the only problem facing the people when it comes to the delivery of health care. Other, equally important, problems are the maldistribution of health manpower, the unequal access to services, the unreliable quality of care, and the lack of public control over health care. No matter how much we guarantee the payment of services to the people, it is of little comfort to them if there is no one around to provide the service.

And finally, in 1990, perhaps the most prominent of a spate of reports and program proposals for health-care reform issued that year had this to say (Pepper Commission, 2):

"The American health care system is approaching a breaking point. Rapidly rising medical costs are increasing the numbers of people without health coverage and straining the system's capacity to provide care for those who cannot pay. The gap is widening between the majority of Americans, who can take advantage of the best medical services in the world, and the rest, who find it hard to get even basic needed care. As the gap increases, the weight of financing care for those without adequate coverage is undermining the stability of our health care institutions. Even for the majority, the explosive growth in health care costs is steadily eroding the private insurance system—the bulwark they count on as their defense against financial risk in case of illness. Perhaps Senator David Durenberger of Minnesota said it best (Pepper Commission, 2): "The American health care system . . . [is] a paradox of plenty and want. . . .""

On the other hand, some observers deny that any serious problems exist other than those brought on by the reformers themselves. In 1972, in his book *The Case for American Medicine*, journalist Harry Schwartz, Ph.D., wrote that cries of "crisis" were just so much hyperbole: U.S. medicine has been doing an outstanding job, and new research and sociological change is needed to improve the nation's health further *(American Medical News)*. In his ongoing series of articles in the "throwaway" journal *Private Practice*, Dr. Schwartz continued to hold this view into the 1990s.

In 1990, writing in *Private Practice*, Dr. Edward Annis, who as the President of the American Medical Association at the time led that organization's fight against the enactment of Medicare, agreed with Dr. Schwartz's view: "So-called experts claim that the United States faces a health-care crisis (October)." "Americans are blessed with the world's finest medical-care system. . . . The U.S. system is superior to all others. . . .[I]t was the government that drove a wedge between doctors and their patients (January)."

The Present Situation

Most current observers, however, have taken the position that we continue to face serious problems and they are getting worse. Costs have continued to rise. As noted above, in 1988, $540 billion was spent for health care, 11.1 percent of the gross national product. The corresponding figures for 1960, 1970, and 1980 were $27 billion, 5.3 percent; $75 billion, 7.6 percent; $248 billion, 9.4 percent (USDHHS, 137, Table 72). As of 1987, about 14 percent of Americans, almost 33 million people, lacked health insurance coverage of any kind (*Stat.*, Table 152).

Hospital beds were still maldistributed, with an oversupply of beds in voluntary and proprietary hospitals in many parts of the country and undersupply of beds in public general hospitals in many cities. There was a problem with physician oversupply in certain of the procedure-based specialities while the onward march of physician specialization continued unabated. The medical education system was seen as in serious difficulty (GPEP).

For some observers, the possible rationing of health services was a major concern (Fuchs; Levinsky; Wennberg). There were deficiencies in the quality of medical care and in the measures designed to control quality (IOM). There was a continuing tendency, particularly among teaching hospital–based physicians, to stress the unusual at the expense of the commonplace, to focus on patients with acute physical problems at the expense of patients who are chronically ill or have

mental problems, and to emphasize treatment rather than prevention (Jonas). Finally, several different public opinion surveys done in
the 1980s showed that upwards of 75 percent of the people believed
that the health-care system is in need of major overhaul (Blendon;
Blendon & Altman).

Few if any of these problems with our health-care system are new.
They have simply undergone gradual changes in size. Indeed, many
of the major problems considered by the Committee on the Costs of
Medical Care (1932) and still pressing today originated in our country
and those of our European forebears in the seventeenth, eighteenth,
and nineteenth centuries (Freymann, 3–97). The problems are not
only long-standing; they are embedded in the fabric of American
society.

As stated above, we do not, by definition, face a "health-care crisis."
This fact should not be cause for complacency, however. As modern
medical practice itself illustrates, it is often easier to deal with a
crisis, even a major one, than with chronic problems.

Looking Ahead

A major cause of the problems of the U.S. health-care system is its
highly permissive and pluralistic character. The political, economic,
and social environment created by the Reagan administration in the
1980s has only intensified them. A special aspect of its ideology has
been to encourage privatization of the health-care system (Salmon).
An increasing number of voluntary hospitals have been bought out
by commerical hospital chains. Voluntary and even public hospitals have been turned over to management by private corporations in the expectation that this will enhance efficiency and productivity. Up to this writing, evidence of such effects has not been
demonstrated.

To stem the tide of rising medical and hospital costs, major reliance has been on promoting "competition" in the health-care system. However, for competition to be effective in lowering prices and
improving quality, the consumer must have some reasonable knowledge of what he is buying. Furthermore, he must make most of the
purchases. In health care, consumers know virtually nothing about
what they are buying, and it is the sellers, not the consumers, who
make the majority of the decisions about what shall be purchased at
which price in any case.

National Health Insurance (NHI), by its very name, means government participation at one or more jurisdictional levels throughout

the country in the health-care financing system. NHI proposals have been on the national political agenda with more or less attention paid to them since Teddy Roosevelt made NHI one of the planks of his Bull Moose Party platform in the presidential election of 1912. In the 1980s, NHI faded almost completely from the health-care political agenda. In the 1990s, it is experiencing a revival. Chapter 8 reviews the history of NHI in the United States.

All this means more deliberate planning of the U.S. health-care system to improve the quantity and quality of services and more rational regulation to promote quality and avert abuse. The World Health Organization goal of "Health for All by the Year 2000" should certainly be attainable in the United States. The heterogeneity and pluralism of the U.S. health culture will certainly not vanish, but organization and coordination will enable it to achieve harmonious performance and equity in the years ahead.

REFERENCES

Adams, P. F., & Hardy, A. M. "Current Estimates from the National Health Interview Survey." *Vital and Health Statistics*, Series 10, No. 173, October 1989.

AHA, American Hospital Association. *Hospital Statistics, 1990–1991 Edition*. Chicago, 1990.

American Medical News. "The Case for American Medicine. Chapter II: What Health Crisis? From the New Book by Harry Schwartz." *American Medical News, 1*, 1972.

Annis, E. R. "Freedom Once Was the Key to Quality Medical Care . . ." *Private Practice*, January 1990, p. 16.

Annis, E. R. "Heritage Health Plan Makes Sense." *Private Practice*, October 1990, p. 12.

Battistella, R., & Southby, R. "Crisis in American Medicine." *The Lancet*, March 16, 1968, p. 581.

Blendon, R. J., "Three Systems: A Comparative Study." *Health Management Quarterly*, First Quarter, 1989, p. 2.

Blendon, R. J., & Altman, D. C. "Public Attitudes about Health Care Costs." *New England Journal of Medicine, 311*, 613, 1984.

Committee on the Costs of Medical Care. *Medical Care for the American People*. Chicago: University of Chicago Press, 1932; reprinted, Washington, D.C.: USDHEW, 1970.

Dellums, R. "The Health Service Act: H.R. 2969." *Congressional Record, 125*, (33), 1979.

Fortune Magazine Editors. *Our Ailing Medical System: It's Time to Operate*. New York: Harper & Row, 1970.

Freymann, J. G. *The American Health Care System: Its Genesis and Trajectory.* New York: Medcom Press, 1974.

Fuchs, V. R. "The 'rationing' of Medical Care." *New England Journal of Medicine, 311,* 1572, 1984.

GPEP: General Professional Education of the Physician Panel. "Physicians for the Twenty-First Century." *Journal of Medical Education, 59* (11) (plus appendices), 1–208, 1984.

Grove, R. D., & Hetzel, A. M. *Vital Statistics Rates in the United States: 1940–1960,* Washington, DC: National Center for Health Statistics, USDHEW, 1968.

Hilts, P. J. "Life Expectancy for Blacks in U.S. Shows Sharp Drop." *The New York Times,* November 29, 1990, p. A1.

IOM, Institute of Medicine, Lohr, K. N., ed. *Medicare: A Strategy for Quality Assurance,* Vols. 1, 2. Washington, DC: National Academy Press, 1990.

Jonas, S. "Health Promotion in Medical Education." *American Journal of Health Promotion, 3,* 37, 1988.

Klaw, S. *The Great American Medicine Show.* New York: Viking, 1975.

Levinsky, N. C. "The Doctor's Master." *New England Journal of Medicine, 311,* 1573, 1984.

MVSR, *Monthly Vital Statistics Report.* "Advance Report of Final Mortality Statistics, 1988," Vol. 39, No. 7, Supplement, November 28, 1990.

Office of National Cost Estimates. "National health expenditures, 1988." *Health Care Financing Review,* Summer, 1990, *11,* No. 4, p. 1.

Pepper Commission. *A Call for Action,* Executive Summary. Washington, DC: Government Printing Office, September, 1990.

Research and Policy Committee. *Building a National Health-Care System.* New York: Committee for Economic Development, 1973.

Rogatz, P. "The Health Care System: Planning." *Hospitals,* April 16, 1970, p. 47.

Salmon, J. W., *The Corporate Transformation of Health Care.* Amityville, NY: Baywood, 1990.

Schwartz, E., et al. "Black/White Comparisons of Deaths Preventable by Medical Interventions." *International Journal of Epidemiology, 19,* 591, 1990.

Schwartz, H. *The Case for American Medicine: A Realistic Look at Our Health Care System.* New York: David McKay, 1972.

USDHEW, U.S. Department of Health Education and Welfare. *National Guidelines for Health Planning (Draft).* Washington, DC: Health Resources Administration, 1979.

U.S. Department of Health and Human Services. *Health United States, 1984.* USDHHS Pub. No. (85)–1232. Washington, DC: Government Printing Office, 1984.

Wennberg, J. E. "Outcomes Research, Cost Containment, and the Fear of Health Care Rationing." *The New England Journal of Medicine, 323,* 1202, 1990.

Chapter 2

Primary and Ambulatory Care

PRIMARY CARE

Primary care and ambultory care go together like apple pie and ice cream.* This is so even though not all primary care is delivered in an ambulatory setting, nor is all ambulatory care primary care. Nevertheless, since they are so closely associated, we cover them in the same chapter.

Primary care has proved difficult to define precisely. In 1977 the Institute of Medicine cataloged 33 definitions of primary care (Ruby). In our view, several of them must be combined for a thorough understanding of the concept. As pointed out in Chapter 1, in *ideal*, that is comprehensive, primary care, an appropriately trained health professional or team provides most of the personal preventive and curative care for an individual or family over a significant period. The primary caregiver integrates and explains the patient's or family's overall health problems and needs for care, giving adequate attention to their psychological and social dimensions, and coordinates any services to be sought from other health professionals. In *functional* terms, primary care is that care most people need most of the time for most of their health concerns.

The central aspect of comprehensive primary care is its integrating role. When nearly all medical services were rendered by a family's general practitioner, coordination was almost automatic. Today, a primary-care doctor or team can still provide most of the care that is necessary most of the time. Complications or new problems will at times, however, require the expertise of others. Coordination can be

---

*For consideration of health manpower in primary care, see Chapter 4.

assured if the primary provider assesses the situation, helps the patient with a proper referral, and then integrates the outcome of the referral into the patient's ongoing care. This "gatekeeper" function of the primary provider prevents fragmentation and the hit-or-miss nature of self-referral to subspecialists (Somers). As White (1973, p. 362) so splendidly put it some years ago: "One wants to avoid the confusion inherent in the encounter between the patient who implicitly says to the doctor, 'I hope you treat what I've got' and the physician who implicitly says to the patient, 'I hope you've got what I treat.'" Another important aspect of the integrating role of comprehensive primary care is the coordination of preventive and curative services. This occurs less often than it should in much American clinical practice.

In contrast to the situation in many other countries, the primary-care relationship in the United States does not end at the hospital admitting office. U.S. primary-care physicians provide a good deal of the inpatient care. Most board-certified family practitioners, general internists, and general pediatricians in this country have hospital admitting privileges. In most other industrialized nations, primary-care physicians work only in offices and health centers; a separate group of specialists provides inpatient and hospital clinic care. Unfortunately, many people in the United States do not have access to comprehensive primary care but receive fragmented outpatient and inpatient services, often only after they become seriously ill.

The primary-care concept is not new. It received strong support from the Committee on the Costs of Medical Care in the 1930s and other authorities in the intervening years (Somers). In Great Britain, the concept goes back at least as far as the Dawson report of 1920 on the structure of health services (Sidel & Sidel, p. 152). In the United States, as physician specialization and subspecialization increased dramatically in the period following World War II, much of the ambulatory care provided in private offices and groups and in hospital outpatient departments became highly fragmented (Freymann, p. 152). The need to restore continuity and coordination was recognized in the 1960s and led to a revitalization of the concept of primary care (Institute of Medicine). Many neighborhood health centers developed in the 1960s and 1970s fostered the primary-care approach, as did many health maintenance organizations developed in the 1970s and 1980s (see below).

As noted above, primary care is not limited to ambulatory care, but ambulatory care is central to primary care. If primary care is to become a major function for physicians, ambulatory care too will have to become a major function of physicians and of the institutions that train them.

AMBULATORY CARE

Ambulatory care is personal health service given to a person who is not a bed patient in a health-care institution.* The term thus covers all health services other than community health services and personal health services for the institutionalized patient. The majority of physician-patient contacts in the United States occur in an ambulatory setting.

There are two principal categories of ambulatory care. The largest is that given by private physicians in solo, partnership, or private group practice on a fee-for-service basis. The other is that provided in organized settings. The latter is defined as a locus of medical practice with an identity independent from that of the individual physician working in it. This category includes hospital-based ambulatory services, (e.g., clinics, emergency departments, health promotion centers); emergency medical services systems such as those run by police and fire departments; free-standing "emergi-centers" and "surgi-centers"; health department clinics; neighborhood health centers (NHCs), and community health centers (CHCs); health maintenance organizations (HMOs); organized home care; community mental health centers; industrial health services; school health services; prison health services. Unfortunately, there is not space to cover all of these categories.

Utilization

In 1988 about 9.5 times as many people contacted a physician in person on an ambulatory basis or by phone as were admitted to a hospital (Adams & Benson, Table D): About 77 percent of the population made at least one physician contact, and about 8 percent of the population was hospitalized one or more times. Overall, Americans averaged 4.8 physician visits per person annually, excluding telephone contacts but including inpatient visits (Adams & Benson, Table 71), about the same as in 1981.

---

*In 1981 Dr. M. I. Roemer published a comprehensive review of the subject, *Ambulatory Health Services in America*.

Utilization of ambultory care varies with age, sex, region, and income (Adams & Benson, Table 71). During 1989, the frequency of physician visits increased with patient age after the age of 5 from an average of 2.2 office visits per year for children 5–17 to 6.0 visits per year for people 75 and over. Females had one more visit per year than males (3.7 to 2.7). The office-visit rate by region ranged from 3.4 in the South to 3.1 in the Midwest and West.

White people had over one more office visit per year than blacks (3.4 to 2.3; Adams & Benson, Table 71). In 1981, the visit rates by ethnic group were virtually the same (USDHHS, 1984, p. 97). Thus a equalization trend which had been under way since 1964 was reversed. It is possible, although certainly not proven, that this "visit gap" has something to do with the observed widening gap between white and black mortality rates noted in the previous chapter.

On the other hand, an equalization of visit rates over time by income was maintained (Adams & Benson, Table 71). Among families earning less than $10,000 in 1989, the office-visit utilization rate was 3.4, compared with 3.3 for those earning $35,000. In 1964, the physician visit rate for the under-$7,000 group (a much larger one in those days) was 3.9, compared with 5.2 for the over-$25,000 group (USDHHS, 1984, p. 97).

The causes of these changes are unclear. They may be related in part to the availability of Medicaid coverage to some of the poor in some states, which could increase utilization for those with that coverage. They may be due in part to rising out-of-pocket costs for the insured and self-payers, which could decrease utilization for those with that coverage. It is important to note that medical care used does not necessarily reflect the extent to which health needs are met.

Hospital Outpatient Departments

The institutional center of the American health-care system is the hospital (see Chapter 3). For a variety of historical reasons, most American hospitals focus the bulk of their efforts and activities on *inpatients*, who are acutely ill and confined to bed (Freymann, chap. 3). Hospitals also have had to deal with a variety of other types of patients, however. Among them are those not requiring immediate admission to a bed, known as *outpatients*.

Hospital outpatients require either immediate treatment for an acute and often serious illness or injury or ongoing care for a more routine matter. Very often the services of the latter type are similar to those needed by patients who attend private practitioners' offices. In theory at least, there are two categories of hospital ambulatory services, corresponding to the two categories of patient needs: emergency services, provided by emergency rooms or departments, and clinic services. In the real world, overlap between the two categories of patient and service is increasing. Patients, hospital staffs, and administrations are sometimes confused about the differences in role and function of the two divisions. All three sometimes have trouble deciding who should go where for what.

It has been easier for hospitals to determine that emergency services should be provided than that clinic services should be. One reason for this is that insurance carriers are more likely to reimburse hospitals for emergency services than for clinic services. Over 80 percent of U.S. hospitals have emergency units (AHA, Table 12A). The original intended functions of emergency units were to take care of people acutely ill or injured, particularly with life-threatening or potentially life-threatening problems that required immediate attention, personnel, and/or equipment not found in private practitioners' offices, and to offer the availability of prompt hospitalization if needed. Most hospitals have found it desirable or necessary (legally required in some states) to provide such services.

On the other hand, with a few exceptions only two kinds of hospitals provide broad-based medical and surgical clinic services, corresponding to the services provided by private physicians in their offices. First are those located in areas where patients could not or would not attend private practitioners' offices for more routine care, usually for economic reasons (Roemer, 1971, 1981). Second are those that have teaching programs. Although it has done so in the past, the American Hospital Association no longer reports the number of hospitals providing broad-based clinic services.

Historical Background

In the nineteenth century, clinic service was part of the function of most hospitals serving the poor in urban areas (Freymann, chaps. 3, 4). However, until the late nineteenth century, hospitals were not too common in the United States. In 1875, there were fewer than 200 of them (Stevens, p. 52). A building boom then took place, and by 1909, there were 4,359 hospitals, with a bed capacity of 421,000. Most of these were "voluntary hospitals" (see Chapter 3), established not to make a profit but to provide community service.

By 1916, 495 hospitals had clinics, often serving an educational as well as a charitable function (Roemer, 1981). The original purpose of some of the hospitals built during this period was to provide special services to meet needs brought on by a rapidly changing world. For example, in 1908 the Goshen (New York) Emergency Hospital was established. Its creation was stimulated by the building of one of New York State's early trunk highways, Route 17. The road went through the center of the village. Traffic accidents occurred with increasing frequency, ergo the hospital.

Also during this era, local government hospitals were established for the sole purpose of taking care of the poor, both inpatients and outpatients. The first of these developed from the infirmaries that had been established in the poorhouses-workhouses. The latter provided general custodial functions for persons who were for any reason not self-sufficient.

Both the voluntaries and the local government hospitals provided free clinic care to the poor. Because their medical staffs consisted primarily of physicians practicing privately in the community, the former were much more important in setting the style for the organization of medical practice than the latter. In most cases, the voluntaries established clinics on their premises only grudgingly since they were likely to be used by nonpaying patients. When a clinic was built onto the archetypical nineteenth-century voluntary hospital, the Johns Hopkins in Baltimore, it was added at the back (Freymann, p. 56). As Freymann said (p. 200): "It was and still is an appendix tacked on the periphery of the bed-filled tower that soaks up the pride and wealth of the community. The ambulatory services huddle at the nether end of the pecking order." Nevertheless, many of the medical-school-affiliated voluntaries that established clinics did come to see over time their utility for medical education and research.

Hospital Clinic Organization and Staffing

While not all clinics are found in teaching hospitals (those affiliated with medical schools), they are the archetype. Given the way contemporary medical education is structured, the teaching hospitals found that the best way of organizing outpatient clinics to provide opportunities for teaching and research is to have many disease-, organ-, or organ-system-specific clinics (Freymann, p. 255). Typically the contemporary teaching hospital has three groups of clinics: medical, surgical, and other.

The medical clinics, of which a "general medical clinic" approximating the function of the general-internist or family-practice unit may be a part, include cardiology, neurology, dermatology, allergy, gastroenterology, and so on. Patients may remain under the care of one or more specialty clinics for long periods. This is especially true where the general-medical or family-practice clinic is small or nonexistent and specialty clinics accept patients directly on self- or professional referral.

General surgery, orthopedics, urology, plastic surgery, and the like compose the surgical clinic group. Surgical care is usually more episodic than general medical care. Thus patients are not as likely to remain for long periods under the care of these clinics. Included in the third, "catchall" group are pediatrics and the pediatric subspecialties, obstetrics-gynecology and its subspecialties, and others such as rehabilitation medicine.

There are five functional categories of physician staff in teaching-hospital clinics. First, it was formerly very common for the hospital's "voluntary" attending medical staff to draw clinic duty as part of the obligation incurred for the grant of the privilege to admit and take care of their private patients in the hospital at no cost to themselves ("admitting privileges"). This is still the case in some institutions.

Second, in the 1980s many medical schools became increasingly dependent for their financial support on physician income earned in the clinics. The money is derived primarily from third-party insurers (see Chapter 7). Thus many clinics are now staffed by medical-school faculty whose work there generates both some of their own income and money for the school's general fund. The management system for dividing this income between the physicians and the institution is called the "clinical practice plan." Depending upon the particular arrangements, for some physicians the medical-school hospitals have become more rather than less attractive places to work in.

Third, to carry out teaching, supervisory, and research functions, the hospital may assign full-time salaried inpatient physicians, usually more junior ones, to the clinics. Fourth, house staff (physicians in post–medical-school specialty training) usually draw significant clinic duty from time to time throughout the course of their training. (Since house staff are usually rotated frequently between various subspecialty clinics for teaching purposes, patients with stable conditions coming to a subspecialty clinic, say once every three months, may see a different physician each time.) Finally, for clinics with many patient visits, hospitals may hire outside physicians exclusively to work in them on a sessional or part-time salaried basis.

Most hospital outpatient departments are open all day on weekdays, but many individual clinics, particularly when they are highly subspecialized, meet only once or twice a week. The larger teaching hospitals often have over 100 specialty and subspecialty clinics. Thus, a hospital-based physician working in the usual hosptial-clinic organization can concentrate on diabetes, peripheral vascular disease, or stroke in her or his teaching and/or research. This is useful for the provider focusing on a particular disease or condition. It also may be helpful to the patient who has a single disease or problem of a rather complex or unusual nature. But for other patients, it may not be.

Patient Difficulties in the Clinics

Three kinds of patients face difficulties in using such clinics. First is the patient with the ordinary problem for which no specialty clinic exists; few hospitals have a "sore-throat" clinic. Second is the patient with a categorical disease, like congestive heart failure, which, however, is uncomplicated. Going to a cardiac clinic, such a patient is likely to have to take a backseat to patient who has cardiac disease with complications. Third is the patient with multiple problems. These patients, often elderly, may attend cardiac clinic on Tuesday, renal (kidney) clinic on Wednesday, peripheral vascular disease clinic on Thursday, and diabetes clinic on Friday. This is distinctly disadvantageous, for two reasons. First, the patient must make multiple trips to the hospital. Second, she is much more likely to be seen by the institution as a collection of diseased organ systems rather than a whole person.

The basic contradiction in hospital ambulatory services is clear. On the one hand, there are the teaching and research needs of specialty-oriented providers. On the other, there are the needs of patients with ordinary problems or several problems requiring the care of several specialties. This situation is not new; neither is professional recognition of it and recommendations for correcting it. In 1964, at a conference on "The Expanding Role of Ambulatory Services in Hospitals and Health Departments" held at the New York Academy of Medicine, Cecil Sheps, M.D., said (p. 148):

> As I sat through the sessions yesterday and today I had a persistent feeling of *deja vu*. I possess a book written by Michael M. Davis [*Clinics, Hospitals and Health Centers*, New York: Harper, 1927] and published in 1927. In it there is quoted a statement prepared in 1914 that describes the purpose of an out-patient department just as clearly as anything said at this conference; that the focus must be on the patient, that care must be organized around the patient, and that the hospital must take the community as its venue and not simply the patients who come to it.

At the same conference, John Knowles, M.D., outlined his view of comprehensive ambulatory care in the hospital setting in terms that are still perfectly applicable (p. 73):

> Comprehensive medicine in this [ambulatory care] context means the coordination of all the various caring elements in the community with those of the medical profession by a team of individuals representing all disciplines, with all the techniques and resources available to the physician and his patient. The aim of these individuals would be to provide total care—somatic, psychic, and social—to those in need, and to study and research the expanding social and economic problems of medical care with the intent of improving the organization and provision of health services.

Another version of this vision is John Gordon Freymann's "mission-oriented hospital" (see Chapters 3 and 6). In few hospitals have these objectives been recognized as primary; much less have they been achieved.

The 1990s version of what Dr. Davis was talking about in 1927 is called community-oriented primary care (Madison; Mullan; Mullan & Connor; Nutting). Its major elements are:

1. The clinical practice of comprehensive primary medical care.
2. The use of applied epidemiology in practice planning.
3. Community involvement in program planning.
4. The use of data gathered in practice operations in a feed-back loop.
5. Continuing surveillance of community health status and needs.

The model can be used in any medical practice, whether solo, group, or hospital-based. The principal problem is not conceptual; the ideas have been with us for many years. The difficulty is in implementation.

Hospital Emergency Services

As noted above, more than 80 percent of American hospitals have emergency departments (AHA, Table 12A). In 1989, there were almost 90 million visits made to over 5,000 hospital emergency departments (AHA, Tables 5A, 12A). The hospital emergency unit serves a variety of functions. First, it provides care to critically ill and injured patients. Second, in many hospitals it also serves as a secondary well-equipped private doctor's office. There, staff physicians can see their own patients who require more sophisticated care than that available in the doctor's office. Third, emergency departments are a source of patient admissions to the hospital. An increasingly important fourth role is the provision of care to persons who are not injured or critically ill, but who have not reached or cannot reach a private physician, or find that their clinic is not open when needed.

In terms that still apply, back in 1966, Weinerman et al. (p. 1037) defined three categories of patients presenting themselves to emergency units:

1. *Nonurgent:* Condition does not require the resources of an emergency service; referral for routine medical care may or may not be needed; disorder is nonacute or minor in severity.
2. *Urgent:* Condition requires medical attention within the period of a few hours; there is a possible danger to the patient if medically unattended; disorder is acute but not necessarily severe.
3. *Emergent:* Condition requires immediate medical attention; time delay is harmful to patient; disorder is acute and potentially threatening to life or function.

Of course, these are professional definitions. Many patients do not make these kinds of distinctions. And most visits to emergency rooms are for conditions that are not "urgent" from a medical viewpoint. Nevertheless, most patients presenting themselves for care do so because regardless of how their problem might be classified by a provider, they feel they need attention immediately, and they cannot find appropriate care elsewhere. Whatever the patient's problem, it is distressing to him. However, such patients load emergency departments with responsibilities to which they are not ideally suited.

In the view of many analysts, the solution must he found outside the walls of the hospital. It must encompass an integrated system of medical care for the entire community, ensuring availability of appropriate medical care at all hours and to all classes of the population. Thus we come full circle back to the definitions of comprehensive and community-oriented primary care reviewed at the beginning of this chapter, and to the visions of Michael Davis, John Knowles, and John Gordon Freymann.

Freestanding Emergi-centers

In the 1980s one partial solution to the problem appeared that found favor with some patients in need. On the other hand, according to some authorities, it caused consternation for those hospitals that saw their emergency-department patient census drop because of the new development (Powills). Others felt that the new entity had little effect on hospitals, its impact being more on private physicians' office practice. It is called the *emergi-center* or *urgi-center* (Ermann & Gabel). Freestanding emergency-care centers provide episodic emergency care 24 hours a day, seven days a week. The patient profile is similar to that of hospital emergency rooms. However, since there is no immediate access to major operating rooms, presumably there are fewer patients appearing with life-threatening emergencies.

Urgi-centers are similar to emergi-centers but are not open all the time. Again, presumably (since there are no comprehensive studies of these facilities available) urgi-centers see an even higher proportion of nonurgent patients than emergi-centers do. The most commonly treated conditions are respiratory tract, ear, and urinary tract infections; sprains and fractures; and abdominal pain. Patients may drop in without appointments, and waiting times are usually short. It is estimated that there are several thousand such facilities. Many are physician-owned. However, to deal with the competition, hospitals, especially those in multihospital systems, have entered the business too.

Emergency Medical Services

Emergency medical services are those provided on an immediate basis to victims of accidents and acute overwhelming illnesses. The goal is to preserve life and/or diminish the degree of temporary and/or permanent disability suffered by the victim. Virtually all patients entering the emergency medical services system are in the "emergent" or "urgent" category. Emergency medical services often begin outside the hospital. As pointed out by Ruth Roemer et al. (1975) in a detailed treatment of the history and major problems of this service sector, the emergency medical service (EMS) has three principal components: (1) ambulance services and emergency prehospital care, (2) emergency medical care provided at the hospital, and (3) disaster medical services.

Federal EMS legislation identifies 15 components of a functioning emergency medical services system (Hoffer): provision of labor-force, training of personnel, communications, transportation, facilities, critical-care units, use of public-safety agencies, consumer participation, accessibility to care, transfer of patients, standard medical-record keeping, consumer information and education, independent review and evaluation, disaster linkage, and mutual-aid agreements. A principal goal has been to provide the whole nation with a network of coordinated emergency-care dispatch centers, using the uniform emergency telephone number 911.

Ambulances are the key link. They transport EMS patients safely and quickly to an appropriate emergency medical facility, and at a minimum their personnel provide first aid at the site and in transit (Gibson). Historically, ambulance services developed from a for-profit enterprise established by funeral directors. In this system, sometimes the same vehicle served more than one purpose, on occasion consecutively.

Beginning in the 1970s, specialized, sometimes very highly equipped vehicles manned by well-trained personnel began to make their appearance. Called emergency medical services (EMS), they are now common in certain parts of the country, especially large cities. EMS are seriously deficient in many parts of the United States, although in the 1980s the situation improved somewhat in certain localities, especially those served by volunteer fire and/or ambulance corps. Given that traumatic injury is among the leading causes of death in the productive age groups and that early attention following traumatic injury can often be lifesaving, this state of affairs is particularly disturbing.

Public Health Agency Clinics

At the local level in many parts of the United States, government provides ambulatory personal health services (see also 5). Local health departments operate an array of special clinics, focusing primarily on the prevention of disease. Among local governments, there is a wide variation in the number and type of services offered. Precisely how much care is provided is not known. In 1975 it was estimated that less than 3 percent of all ambulatory personal health services were being provided by local health departments, excluding school health services (M. I. Roemer, 1975). There are over 2,000 local health-department units providing some kind of health service in the United States.

Important among their services are clinics for tuberculosis control (often giving treatment as well as case-detection service), child health (where immunizations, examinations, and education on childrearing are provided), prenatal care, sexually transmitted disease (STD) control, and mental health problems. In recent years, some public health agencies have broadened the scope of their services to include family planning (birth control), chronic disease detection, and in certain locales, general primary care.

The provision of personal disease-treatment service by local health departments has been a subject of controversy ever since the practice began in the nineteenth century (Rosen; Winslow, chap. 17; see also below, Neighborhood Health Centers). Private physicians have generally regarded local health departments as competing for their fee-paying patients and therefore threatening their practices. Since local health departments, in contrast to local hospital departments, traditionally offered their services free to all persons, regardless of ability to pay, this fear was not groundless. Battles over the role of local health departments were especially fierce during the 1920s when some local health departments developed plans to expand their general disease-treatment services (Myers et al.; Rosen; Winslow, chap. 17).

The efforts of the organized representatives of American physicians generally met with success. To this day, most local health department personal services are limited to those areas in which private physicians are either not very interested (routine well-baby examinations) or not especially competent (treatment, case finding, and contact investigation for sexually transmitted disease and tuberculosis). In the current era, there has been a diminution of organized medicine's opposition to the involvement of local health departments in the provision of direct medical services to the poor. Some hard-pressed urban and suburban health departments have done this, especially where there are limited public-hospital services.

Neighborhood and Community Health Centers

In the late 1960s and early 1970s, a phenomenon called the neighborhood health center (NHC) emerged on the American health-care scene. It was based on the concepts of full-time salaried physician staffing, multidisciplinary team health-care practice, and community involvement in both policy-making and facility operations (Davis & Schoen; Zwick). The movement was strongly stimulated by the federal Office of Economic Opportunity (OEO). It was the lead agency for the "war on proverty" conducted by President Lyndon Johnson's administration between 1964 and 1968.

The neighborhood health center movement was a rallying cry, a focus for the way to "do things right." It did not meet with overwhelming success, to say the least. Its successor, the community health center (CHC) system, has entered the 1990s with ever-decreasing federal support but has survived (see the end of this section). The NHC movement did not become a major element in the American health-services landscape in patient visits provided, for example. Ideologically it was very important, however. Its basic concepts have been given continuing vitality in the community-oriented primary care (COPC) model (Mullan & Conner). COPC may receive new life if provision is ever made to provide coverage for those 33 million or so Americans who currently have no health insurance.

The NHC did not represent an entirely new concept in the United

States. The nineteenth-century freestanding urban "dispensary" was an early general ambulatory-care center serving primarily the poor. Although it was organized differently, it performed some functions similar to those of the modern NHC or CHC. Health department ambulatory-care programs developed during the last quarter of the nineteenth century had some elements that would also appear later in NHCs, such as districting. For the most part, however, they provided categorical services and therefore were not comprehensive.

Nevertheless, the period from 1910 to 1919 was marked by the development of several local health centers that truly attempted to offer comprehensive services to designated areas from a freestanding, nonhospital-based institution (Rosen). Winslow noted in 1919: "The most striking and typical development of the public health movement of the present day is the health center" (Rosen). However, he was overoptimistic. During the period from 1920 to 1923, Herman Biggs, M.D., then commissioner of health of New York State, tried vigorously, but quite unsuccessfully, to get the state and local health departments away from the categorical-disease approach and into the business of delivering comprehensive health services (Windslow, chap. 17). As noted above, organized medicine fought hard and with success against any health-care delivery mode not based on private practice (except for service to the very poor).

The experience with prepaid group practice (PPGP) in the 1930s, 1940s, and 1950s influenced the development of the NHC movement of the 1960s and 1970s. For example, the first director of one of the first NHCs, established on New York City's Lower East Side (Light & Brown), Gouverneur, came from one of the prototypical PPGPs, the Health Insurance Plan of Greater New York. Serving as a model that many persons who were establishing NHCs came to observe, Gouverneur was very influential in the early development of OEO-funded NHCs.

NHCs were usually situated in medically underserved urban minority communities. With varying degrees of vigor and success, they attempted to make multidisciplinary group practice work. As well as physicians and nurses, they employed social workers, "neighborhood health workers" (usually people from the area served, specially trained by the NHC with a combination of basic nursing and social service skills), and sometimes lawyers, all on salary. These folks were combined into a health-care team. The NHCs aimed to provide one-stop shopping for comprehensive ambulatory care, a full range of preventive, rehabilitative, and treatment services that were acceptable, affordable, and of high quality. The NHCs also aimed to intervene in the cycle of poverty.

At the movement's peak in the early 1970s, nationally there were an estimated 200 NHCs *(Health PAC Bulletin)*. In the mid-1970s, the Nixon and Ford administrations more narrowly defined the scope of the NHC program and renamed it the community health center program. The CHCs, which included many of the original NHCs, were to concentrate on the delivery of primary-care services. They were to deemphasize other NHC roles, such as providing employment opportunities and training programs, stimulating social and economic development in their communities, and concerning themselves with environmental as well as personal health problems.

By the early 1980s, there were over 800 CHCs serving over 4.5 million people (Sardell), a remarkable resurgence for a program that received little publicity. The CHCs were supported primarily by federal grants, third-party reimbursements, and private fees paid on a sliding scale. Following a comprehensive review of available utilization data, Freeman et al. (p. 264) concluded:

1. CHCs do provide access to ambulatory health services to residents of low-income and minority areas with a frequency/cost profile approximating that of private medical practice, and typically lower than the costs of care in hospital ambulatory clinics and emergency rooms.
2. CHCs considerably reduced the patient populations of hospital ambulatory clinics and emergency rooms, thus lowering costs.
3. CHC patient populations have measurably lower hospital utilization rates than outpatient hospital-user populations. This was not accounted for by favorable patient "at-risk" selection.

As of 1990, there were about 550 federally supported CHCs operating at over 1500 sites, serving about 5.3 million people, of whom over 60 percent were minority-group members and of whom 60 percent had incomes under the poverty level (HRSA). However, given the climate for federal domestic spending in the 1990s, the future of the CHC program must be considered uncertain.

Industrial Health Service Units

The number of "in-plant" health units in the United States is not known, but there are thousands of them. Their degree of development varies widely by plant size and tasks. In small plants (less than 100 workers), health services are ordinarily rudimentary. They are often limited to a first-aid box and arrangements with some community health facility to which injured workers may be sent. Very large plants (more than 2,500 workers) usually have some systematic in-plant health service. Customarily it is staffed with trained industrial nurses and part-time or full-time physicians.

There is a wide range of industrial health hazards, from traumatic injury to occupational exposure to harmful substances (e.g., silica, asbestos, lead poisoning). In a few firms, in-plant health services are comprehensive, providing employees with complete medical care for all disorders, whether or not job-connected.

The long-term trend in American industry is toward the greater concentration of production in fewer large corporations. This tendency has doubtless led to many economic and social problems. Furthermore, while at one time it seemed that concentration might enhance the prospects for improving occupational health programs, in the latter half of the 1980s, there were actually reductions in service in many large corporations in the name of cost savings (Parkinson).

A relatively recent development in occupational health is the "worksite health promotion" program (Scofield). Of the 50,000 or so firms in the United States that employ over 100 workers, about 12,000 have some kind of health-promotion program (Kamen, 1990). Of those, over 700 have a fitness facility. According to Terborg (p. 225):

> Worksite health promotion consists of an ongoing series of activities funded or endorsed by the organization that are designed to promote the adoption of personal behavior and corporate practices that are conducive to employee fitness, health, and wellness (references). Instruction [and often the opportunity/facility to engage in the activity] is typically provided at the worksite in areas such as exercise, strength training, weight loss, smoking cessation, stress management, blood pressure monitoring and control, and nutrition.

There is some evidence that the provision of such services by companies is cost-effective (Kamen, 1987; Opatz; Shephard).

School Health Clinics

In 1990 there were over 59 million students in about 87,000 primary and secondary schools and colleges and universities (USBoC, Tables 207, 225, 256). Almost all of the educational institutions provide some type of organized ambulatory health service. About one-half of the school health services are run by local health departments, the balance being run by boards of education, on their own (25%) or in cooperation with the local health department. Very little disease treatment is done in school health programs. The work of most is confined to case finding to prevent chronic or epidemic disease (e.g., screening for vision and hearing difficulties and inadequate immunization). This work is done by school nurses; referrals are made to physicians for diagnosis and treatment.

Voluntary Agency Clinics

For many years, voluntary health agencies focusing on special disorders such as tuberculosis, cancer, heart disease, poliomyelitis, and so on have operated clinics. Most of these are run by national associations with numerous local branches. Many were originally formed to sponsor clinics. In the current era, they are more likely to stress the support of medical research and professional education. Some voluntary agencies, however, still operate clinics, such as those for cancer detection sponsored by the American Cancer Society.

In the 1960s, a new type of nongovernmental clinic was started in many large American cities—the "free clinic." These units were usually initiated by youth groups with strong antiestablishment policies. They chose not to use hospital OPDs or public health clinics, which they regarded as too bureaucratic. Instead, the people would raise money to rent a storefront and purchase supplies. They obtained professional services on a voluntary basis from doctors, nurses, pharmacists, and others. For a time, some free clinics even came to be subsidized by local governments. In recent years, many of the free clinics have closed down, but some have become sponsored by established agencies, including medical schools. Other similar "self-help" clinics are sponsored by feminist groups or groups devoted to holistic medicine.

Group Medical Practice

While solo private practice is the predominant mode of organization for physicians in the United States, there has been a gradual trend toward group medical practice. This has taken various forms: private group medical practice, prepaid group practice, health maintenance organizations, independent practice associations (IPA) (in which income, but neither space nor work, is shared), and the latest development, "managed care."

At least five elements of medical practice can be grouped and shared: space, supporting staff, practice income, practice expenditures, and the medical work. Many of the possible permutations and combinations of these elements appear in various forms in the U.S. health-care system. We have space only to scratch the surface.

The American Medical Association defines *group medical practice* as three or more physicians working together and sharing their earnings in some way, regardless of the details of the organizational form. In 1990, there were about 114,000 physicians working in various types of group practices (American Medical Association). Some of them work part-time in more than one group, filling about 150,000 medical "slots" in group practices.

Private Group Medical Practice

In private group medical practice, physicans in private practice share space and often the use and costs of nursing and clerical staff. The group's members bill their patients and/or the patients' insurers individually on the usual fee basis for each service provided. Some groups pool some or all of the income and then pay their members on a partnership basis. In others, the members pay fees to the group from their patient billings to cover common group operations.

Private groups may be single-specialty or multispecialty. Single-specialty groups are common in surgery, anesthesia, and radiology, and are found in increasing numbers in the medical specialties. In this way the responsibilities for round-the-clock coverage can be shared. There are some private multispecialty groups, but these are less common. The major advantages of private group medical practice for physicians are the ability to engage allied health personnel to an extent not feasible for the solo practitioner, the sharing of coverage responsibilities for nights and weekends, and ready access to informal consultations when faced with a difficult diagnostic or therapeutic problem.

Prepaid Group Practice (PPGP)

This form of practice first arose on a very limited basis in the 1890s (Mayer & Mayer). It took the then-revolutionary step of linking a method of payment for medical care in advance of the medical care itself. In conventional health insurance, (see Chapter 7), the insurance company collects money (usually called premiums) from its beneficiaries (in most cases the beneficiaries' employers). It then pays for all or part of the care the beneficiary obtains from the sources of care she uses.

In a PPGP, the organization providing the medical care also acts as the health insurance company for those to whom it provides care. Furthermore, unlike many straight health insurance companies, it provides all or most of the health service required at no additional cost to the patient. As the *Harvard Law Review* said some time ago

(p. 901): "Pre-paid group practice may be broadly defined as a medical care delivery system which accepts responsibility for the organization, financing, and delivery of health services for a defined population."

The two modern major pioneers in this field were the Health Insurance Plan (HIP) in New York City and Kaiser-Permanente on the West Coast. They both took off after the end of World War II. They encountered much resistance from organized medicine (i.e., the American Medical Association and the state and country medical societies). The resistance was based primarily on an antipathy to the way these groups paid their physicians. One method was straight salary. The other was "capitation," that is, paying a flat fee to a primary-care physician to provide a stipulated range of services for the patient for a given time, usually a year. Under capitation, the fee is the same, regardless of how much or little care the patient needs or uses. Both methods were antithetical to the common fee-for-service piecework system used by most American physicians.

Furthermore, organized medicine objected because physicians were no longer independent contractors with their patients. The patients (or their employers) contracted with the PPG to provide the medical care, and that organization contracted with the doctors. For organized medicine, that meant a "loss of control." In a "staff model" PPG, the physicians work on a salaried basis. In the "group model," the physicians join together to form their own company, which in turn contracts with the prepaid group to provide medical services. In this case, the physicians' group pays its individual members on a salary or capitation basis.

As Silver noted many years ago, there are many advantages to PPGP. For the physicians, they include a regular work schedule, guaranteed (although not high) income, a fringe-benefit package including malpractice insurance, the opportunity for collegial medical practice, better access to ancillary personnel and services, and freedom from concern with the business aspects of medical practice. For the patients, the advantages include no or low charges at time of service; one-stop shopping for 24-hour, seven-day service; continuity of care; and protection against unnecessary hospitalization and surgery. The primary disadvantages for patients center around the development of a clinic atmosphere, long delays for service, and impersonality.

The most serious problems with PPGP seem to be that they often do not achieve their potential for improving the practice of medicine. Weinerman, an early strong advocate of prepaid group practice, reviewed the experience in 1968 and was disappointed. His observations, although made some time ago, still apply to many current HMOs and managed-care systems (see below). The organizational advantages for the physicians have been implemented, but clinical medicine remains largely a matter for individual practice. "Group conferences," he said, "medical audits and informal office consultations are, in my experience, more common in the descriptive literature than in daily practice." He concluded (p. 1429):

> Perhaps most disappointing has been the hesitation on the part of most medical groups to effect changes in the "way of life" of the medical team itself. This would involve acceptance by the group as a whole of collective responsibility for the health of its patients or members . . . would mean actively reaching out into the community for . . . early detection . . . [and] identification and special protection for those at specific risk of disease . . . [and] would imply particular concern for those patients who do not use the service. . . . It implies as much concern with rapport as with diagnostic labels, as much with education as prescription.

Once again, the ethic of reform is comprehensive primary care. Once again, it remains to be achieved.

Health Maintenance Organizatons

The health maintenance organization (HMO) movement was originally sponsored by the first Nixon administration. It was interested in the idea because health-services research had revealed that PPGP could save significant amounts of money by reducing hospitalization (Roemer & Schonick). The HMO concept had several variants. One was nothing more or less than PPGP. It happened that in attacking PPGP over the years, organized medicine had liberally red-baited it. Thus, if a Republican administration were to undertake the project, a new name had to be found. The term *health maintenance organization* was invented for Mr. Nixon in the early 1970s by Dr. Paul Ellwood.

HMOs have four major defining characteristics (Thorpe et al.):

1. They assume contractual responsibility for assuring the delivery of a stated range of health care services, including at least inpatient hospital and ambulatory-care services.
2. They serve a voluntarily enrolled population (usually an employee group).
3. The premium is fixed, regardless of utilization. (There may be some small extra charges [co-payments] for the use of certain services.)
4. The HMO assumes some of the financial risk or gain.

One major difference between an HMO and PPGP is that the HMO undertakes to provide or arrange for patient hospitalization when necessary, and those costs are included in the premium paid by the subscriber (acutally most often the subscriber's employer). HMOs have a significant opportunity to integrate health-promotive–disease-preventive services into clinical practice. There is wide variation among the HMOs on the extent or effectiveness with which this is done.

In addition to the staff and group models of physician organization in HMOs, there is also the independent practice association (IPA). It combines solo or small private group practice for the physicians with a prepayment system for the patients. The IPA, like group HMOs, operates a central billing and collection system, peer review for quality and utilization of care, and cost-containment mechanisms.

Until the advent of the Reagan administration, the development of HMOs was supported to some extent by federal subsidies. By 1989, there were over 32 million people enrolled in over 600 HMOs of various types *(Medical Benefits)*. More than 40 percent were in IPAs (which accounted for over 60% of the plans), over 55 percent in plans with more than 100,000 members, about 53 percent in plans which were 10 or more years old, about half in for-profit plans (over 67% of the plans were for-profit), half in not-for-profit plans. Among the developments being undertaken by HMOs as they prepare to meet the challenges of the 1990s are (Belodoff):

- "Point of service plans" allowing members to use nonplan providers by paying an additional fee.
- Increasing cooperation between HMOs and major health insurers like Blue Cross.
- Acceptance of workers-compensation cases.
- Expansion of health-promotion–disease-prevention, worksite-safety, and employees assistance programs (EAPs serve employees with addictive behavior problems).
- Development of packages focused on the currently uninsured population should a comprehensive national health program be instituted (see Chapter 8).

Managed Care

This is the buzzterm of the 1990s in ambulatory care. As Peter D. Fox tells us (p. 1):

"Managed care" . . . broadly defined, encompasses any measure that, from the perspective of the purchaser of health care, favorably affects the price of services, the site at which the services are received, or their utilization. As such, it represents a continuum—from plans that, for example, do no more than require prior authorization of inpatient stays, to the staff model HMO that employs its doctors and assumes risk for delivering a comprehensive benefit package. Ideally managed care should not simply seek to *reduce costs;* rather, it should strive to *maximize value,* which includes a concern with quality and access.

It is interesting to note that managed care is defined *from the perspective of the purchaser* of health care (most often the employer, who is paying the bulk if not all of the health-care premium), not from the perspective of the provider or the patient.

There are a number of forms of managed care (Davis):

• Health maintenance organization.
• Preferred provider organization (PPO): a group of independent providers (usually private practitioners or private medical groups) who have contracted with an insurer to provide named services at fixed fees. (Unlike most IPAs, which are also organizations of privately practicing physicians, the PPO does not focus on the provision of primary care/comprehensive care, but is used more commonly for physicians providing diagnostic and therapeutic invasive procedures.) The fees are set below the prevailing market rate. The insurer's beneficiaries are given a list of the "preferred providers." While the patient does not have to choose a provider from the list, she is guaranteed that there will be no or low copayments if she does so. The advantage to the insurer is cost saving, to the provider a guarantee of work.
• Exclusive provider organization (EPO): similar to the PPO, except that the beneficiary must choose a physician on the insurer's list if he is to receive any reimbursement for the costs of care.
• Independent practice association.
• Independent practice organization (IPO): similar to an IPA, but whereas in IPAs the physicians deal with one insurer, in an IPO the organized group of independently practicing physicians accepts patients and payments from more than one insurer.
• Hospital-physician organization/combined provider organization (HPO/CPO): a variant of the PPO/EPO/IPA/IPO concept organized by a hospital and/or its medical staff. There are many possible combinations of insurance mechanisms, administrative forms, benefit packages, use of copayment, and means of physician and institutional reimbursement.

- "Point of service" plans: variant of all of the above arrangements which allow their beneficiaries some use of providers who are outside of the organization. It is similar to the PPO concept, except that these plans usually attempt to provide a comprehensive package of benefits.

CONCLUSION

The bulk of the need for medical care and the provision of care is in the ambulatory setting. In the United States, a disproportionate share of health-care resources are devoted to inpatient care, both acute and long-term. Given the current profile of disease and disability in the United States, it is obvious that significant improvements in the health of the American people could be achieved by the widespread implementation of known health-promotive–disease-preventive measures in the ambulatory setting (USDHHS, 1990). This is the central element of comprehensive primary care. As stated at the outset of this chapter, primary care goes with ambulatory care like ice cream with apple pie (neither of which is unhealthy if eaten occasionally). Historically, there is movement in the right direction. Much remains to be done.

REFERENCES

Adams, P. F., & Benson, V. "Current Estimates from the National Health Interview Survey." *Vital and Health Statistics*, Series 10, No. 176, October 1990.

AHA, American Hospital Association. *Hospital Statistics: 1990–91*, Chicago: 1989.

American Medical Association. *Medical Groups in the U.S.—a Survey of Practice Characteristics, 1990 Edition.* Chicago: 1990.

Belodoff, H. "HMOs—New Challenges—New Products." In National Health Lawyers Association, *The Insider's Guide to Managed Care*, Washington, DC: 1990.

Davis, G. S. "Introduction: Managed Health Care Primer." In National Health Lawyers Association, *The Insider's Guide to Managed Care.* Washington, DC: 1990.

Davis, K., and Schoen, C., *Health and the War on Poverty.* Washington, DC: The Brookings Institution, 1978.

Ermann, D., & Gabel, J. "The Changing Face of American Health Care: Multihospital Systems, Emergency Centers, and Surgery Centers." *Medical Care, 23,* 401, 1985.

Fox, P. D. "Foreword: Overview of Managed Care Trends." In National Health Lawyers Association, *The Insider's Guide to Managed Care.* Washington, DC: 1990.

Freeman, H. E., et al. "Community Health Centers: An Initiative of Enduring Utility." *Health and Society, 60,* 245, 1982.

Freymann, J. G. *The American Health Care System: Its Genesis and Trajectory.* New York: Medcom Press, 1974.

Gibson, G. "Evaluative Criteria for Emergency Ambulance Services." *Social Science and Medicine, 7,* 425, 1973.

Harvard Law Review. "The Role of Prepaid Group Practice in Relieving the Medical Care Crisis," *84,* 887, 1971.

Health PAC Bulletin. "NENA: Community Control in a Bind," June, 1972.

HRSA, Health Resources and Services Administration. *A Profile.* Washington, DC: U.S. Public Health Service, April 1990.

Hoffer, E. P. "Emergency Medical Services, 1979." *New England Journal of Medicine, 301,* 1118, 1979.

Institute of Medicine. *A Manpower Policy for Primary Health Care.* Washington, DC: National Academy of Sciences, 1978.

Kamen, R. L. "Costs and Benefits of Corporate Health Promotion." *Fitness in Business,* October 1987, p. 39.

Kamen, R. L., American Association of Fitness in Business. Personal communication, October 12, 1990.

Knowles, J. H. "The Role of the Hospital: The Ambulatory Clinic." *Bulletin of the New York Academy of Medicine, 41*(2), 68, 1965.

Light, H. L., & Brown, H. J. "The Gouverneur Health Services Program: An Historical View." *Milbank Memorial Fund Quarterly, 45,* 375, 1967.

Madison, D. L. "The Case for Community-Oriented Primary Care." *Journal of the American Medical Association, 249,* 1279, 1983.

Mayer, T. R., & Mayer, G. G. "HMOs: Origins and Development." *The New England Journal of Medicine, 312,* 590, 1985.

Medical Benefits. "The Interstudy Edge," Vol. 6, No. 11, June 15, 1989, p. 1.

Mullan, F. "Community-Oriented Primary Care." *New England Journal of Medicine, 307,* 1076, 1982.

Mullan, F., & Conner, E., eds. *Community-Oriented Primary Care—Conference Proceedings.* Washington, DC: National Academy Press, 1982.

Myers, B. A., et al. "The Medical Care Activities of Local Health Units." *Public Health Reports, 83,* 757, 1968.

Nutting, P. A., et al. "Community-Oriented Primary Care in the United States." *Journal of the American Medical Association, 253,* 1763, 1985.

Optaz, J. P. *Health Promotion Evaluation,* Steven Point, WI: National Wellness Institute, 1987.

Parkinson, D. Personal communication, October 25, 1990.

Powills, S. "Size of FEC Market a Matter of Opinion." *Hospitals,* May 16, 1985, p. 43.

Roemer, M. I. "Organized Ambulatory Health Service in International Perspective." *International Journal of Health Services, 1,* 18, 1971.

Roemer, M. I. "From Poor Beginnings: The Growth of Primary Care." *Hospitals*, March 1, 1975, p. 38.

Roemer, M. I. *Ambulatory Health Services in America*. Gaithersburg, MD: Aspen Systems, 1981.

Roemer, M. I, & Shonick, W. "HMO Performance: The Recent Evidence." *Health and Society, 51*, 271, 1973.

Roemer, R., et al. *Planning Urban Health Services: From Jungle to System*. New York: Springer Publishing, 1975.

Rosen, G. "The First Neighborhood Health Center Movement—Its Rise and Fall." *American Journal of Public Health, 61*, 1620, 1971.

Ruby, G. "Definitions of Primary Care" (staff paper). Washington, DC: Institute of Medicine, 1977.

Sardell, A. "Neighborhood Health Centers and Community-Based Care: Federal Policy from 1965 to 1982." *Journal of Public Health Policy, 4*, 484, 1983.

Scofield, M. E., ed. *Worksite Health Promotion*. Philadelphia, PA: Hanley & Belfus, 1990.

Shephard, R. J. *Economic Benefits of Enhanced Fitness*. Champaign, IL: Human Kinetics Publishers, 1986.

Sheps, C. G. "Conference Summary and the Road Ahead." *Bulletin of the New York Academy of Medicine, 41*(1), 146, 1965.

Sidel, V. W., & Sidel, R. *A Healthy State*, rev. New York: Pantheon Books, 1983.

Silver, G. A. "Group Practice—What It Is. *Medical Care, 1*, 94, 1963.

Somers, A. R. "And Who Shall be the Gatekeeper? The Role of the Primary Physician in the Health Care Delivery System." *Inquiry, 20*, 301, 1983.

Stevens, R. *American Medicine and the Public Interest*. New Haven, CT: Yale University Press, 1971.

Terborg, J. R. "Health Promotion at the Worksite: A Research Challenge for Personnel and Human Resources Management." *Research in Personnel and Human Resources Management, 4*, 225, 1986.

Thorpe, K. E., et al. "Health Maintenance Organizations." In S. Jonas, ed., *Health Care Delivery in the United States*, 3rd ed. New York: Springer Publishing, 1986.

USBoC, US Bureau of the Census. *Statistical Abstract of the United States: 1990*, (110th edition). Washington, DC.

USDHHS, US Department of Health and Human Services. *Health United States, 1984*. Pub. No. (PHS) 85-1232. Washington, DC: Government Printing Office, 1984.

USDHHS. *Health People 2000*. Washington, DC: Government Printing Office, 1990.

Weinerman, E. R. "Problems and Perspectives of Group Practice." *Bulletin of the New York Academy of Medicine*, 2nd Series, *44*, 1423, 1968.

Weinerman, E. R., et al. "Yale Studies in Ambulatory Medical Care: V. Determinants of Use of Hospital Emergency Services." *American Journal of Public Health, 56*, 1037, 1966.

White, K. L. "Organization and Delivery of Personal Health Services—Public Policy Issues." *Milbank Memorial Fund Quarterly*, January 1968. Reprinted in J. B. McKinlay, ed., *Politics and Law in Health Care Policy.* New York: Prodist, 1973.

Winslow, C. E. A. *The Life of Herman Biggs.* Philadelphia, PA: Lea & Febiger, 1929.

Zwick, D. I. "Some Accomplishments and Findings of Neighborhood Health Centers." *Milbank Memorial Fund Quarterly*, October 1972. Reprinted in I. K. Zola and J. B. McKinlay, eds., *Organizational Issues in the Delivery of Health Services.* New York: Prodist, 1974.

Chapter **3**

Hospitals

The hospital is the institutional center of the health-care system (Knowles). Because of its complexity, the hospital has been described as a city whose major enterprises are the treatment of disease and the restoration of its citizens' health. Like our cities, the hospital has changed dramatically in the past century (Rosenberg). While at the turn of the twentieth century a person entering a hospital had less than a 50 percent chance of leaving it alive, today a patient can expect to benefit from his hospital stay. Typically, 97 percent of patients admitted leave the hospital alive. The hospital has evolved from a place of refuge where a person went to spare his family the anguish of watching him die to a multiservice institution providing interdisciplinary medical care to ambulatory and bed patients.

The modern hospital is also the center of much clinical training, both graduate and undergraduate, for many health professions, and continuing health-sciences education, both formal and informal. In addition, some teaching hospitals are major medical-research institutions. The hospital is the workplace for most U.S. physicians (in addition to their private offices) and at present the only place where they are likely to be subject to peer review of their medical-care performance.

The hospital also has symbolic importance. Being the most visible component of the health-care system, it *is* that system in the minds of many laymen. Its increasingly complex and sometimes bewildering structures and methods have come to represent the growing complexity of the delivery system as a whole.

HISTORICAL DEVELOPMENT

Historically hospitals have been linked with care for the poor with short- or long-term health problems (Stern, chaps. 2, 6; Freymann,

pp. 28–29), and to treatment of the acutely ill of all social classes
(Freymann, pp. 21–29, chap. 4). The word *hospitals* shares its Latin
root with the words *hostel* and *hotel.* Most frequently under church
sponsorship, the institution originated in the Middle Ages as a place
of refuge for the poor, the sick, the just plain weary.

In the European settlements in America, the earliest hospitals were
infirmaries attached to poorhouses. (A poorhouse was an institution
operated by local government to house persons who were un-
employed, orphans or abandoned children, elderly and incapable of
self-care, or mentally ill–retarded.) The first was established at Hen-
ricopolis in Virginia (1612), the next not until 1732 in Philadelphia
(Stern, chap. 6). The first public institution designed solely for the
care of the sick was the "pesthouse" built on Manhattan Island north
of New York City at a place called Belle Vue in 1794. The public
workhouse (also called the poorhouse) was moved to the grounds of
the pesthouse in 1816. It was not until 1848 that New York City
created an independent hospital for the poor by formally separating
the administrations of the two institutions (Freymann, pp. 28–29).
The famous Bellevue Hospital is still in that location.

Nongovernment charity (private "voluntary") hospitals to care for
the poor were first established in the American colonies in the eighteenth century (Freymann, pp. 22–24). (Since hospitals could do little
for their patients, there was no reason for the self-supporting sick to
go to them.) The first one was the Pennsylvania Hospital in Philadelphia, founded by Benjamin Franklin in 1751. By 1873, there
were an estimated 178 hospitals in the United States, many solely for
the mentally ill (Stevens, p. 52). Then a hospital building boom
began.

Over the next few decades, hospitals were built everywhere in
America. By the turn of the twentieth century, a patient admitted to a
general hospital had a better than even chance of getting out alive.
That milestone was achieved largely by the development of general
hospital hygiene, asepsis, and surgical anesthesia. By 1910, general
hospitals had been established in many communities, a total of nearly 4,400, with 421,000 beds (Stevens, p. 52).

The rapid advance of medical science has lead to the expansion of
the hospital system and individual hospitals and their evolution as
the center of the medical-care system (MacEachern, pp. 21–27). After
the turn of the century, medical care quickly became far too complex
for the physician to be able to carry its entire armamentarium in his
black bag. Then the technological capability for intervention in the
disease process quickly became far too complex to carry out at the
side of the patient's bed.

CLASSIFICATION OF HOSPITALS

One major agency that counts and classifies hospitals in the United States is the American Hospital Association (AHA). (The other is the National Center for Health Statistics [NCHS] of the USDHHS, which runs the National Hospital Discharge Survey.) The AHA regularly publishes its *Guide Issue* for the hospital world and the compendium *Hospital Statistics* (AHA, 1990). These publications list each AHA-registered hospital, giving its basic characteristics and much summary data. Mandated by Congress, an annual report to the President entitled *Health: United States* has been published since 1976 (NCHS). It includes data on health status, health resources, and financing. This chapter uses AHA definitions and data, except as specifically noted. The primary ones are

- *Hospital size.* The "average number of beds, cribs, and pediatric bassinets regularly maintained (set up and staffed for use) for inpatients during the reporting period" (AHA, 1990, p. xxii).
- *Hospital type.* There are four: mental, including alcoholism and other chemical dependencies; tuberculosis and other respiratory disease; other special; and general medical and surgical. The "other special" category includes, for example, maternity; eye, ear, nose, and throat; rehabilitation; orthopedic; and chronic disease (AHA, 1990 p. xxi). The "general hospital" category includes the bulk of U.S. hospitals. The AHA has an all-inclusive descriptor for the majority of them: *community hospital,* defined as "all non-federal short term general or other special hospitals, excluding hospital units of institutions [such as prisons and universities] whose facilities and services are available to the public" (AHA, 1990, p. xxi).
- *Mode of ownership.* There are two—private and public. In turn, there are two categories of private hospitals differentiated by the mode of distribution of surplus income: "investor owned," for-profit (proprietary); not-for-profit (voluntary). There are three categories of public hospital, by jurisdiction of ownership: federal, state, and local.
- *Length of stay.* There are two categories: "long" and "short," respectively, 30 days or more, and less than 30 days.

BASIC HOSPITAL DATA

A hospital is usually described by size, type, ownership mode, and predominant length of stay, as well as average daily census (the average number of beds occupied other than by newborns, usually on an annual basis) and occupancy rate (the average proportion of total beds occupied). Table 3.1 presents data on the major classes of hospital. Most common is the voluntary general short-term hospital, followed in number by the local government general short-term hospital. The other major groups are the federal short-term hospitals, the state mental hospitals, and the proprietary short-term hospitals. As of 1990, there were about 1.2 million beds in a total of about 6,700 hospitals, with an average daily census about 850,000 patients and an overall occupancy rate of about 70 percent (AHA, 1990, Table 1).

The hospital profile has changed over time. In 1978, a peak year, there were almost 1.4 million beds in 7,015 hospitals, with an average daily census of 1.04 million patients and an overall occupancy rates of 75.5 percent (AHA, 1979, Tables 1, 2A, 2B). The peak number of community hospitals in the United States, 5,881, was reached in 1977. Between 1964 and 1978, the number of beds increased from 721,000 to 975,000, or 35 percent. During the same period, reflecting the decline in the number of small hospitals, the average number of beds per hospital increased by 32 percent, (AHA, 1979, pp. vii–viii).

TABLE 3.1 Major Hospital Groups, United States, Basic Characteristics

Class:	Federal	Nonfederal mental	Not-for-profit short-term	For-profit short-term	State & local short term
Hospitals	340	741	3,233	769	1,495
Beds (thou.)	101	161	661	102	172
Annual Admis- sions (thou.)	1,811	707	22,798	3,071	5,271
Avg. daily census (thou.)	74	136	455	53	112
Occu- pancy, (percent)	73	84	69	52	65
Avg. length of stay (days)	NA	NA	7.3	6.3	7.7

Source: AHA, 1990, Table 1.

TEACHING HOSPITALS

As used by the AHA, the term *teaching hospital* refers to hospitals providing undergraduate and/or graduate teaching for medical students and/or medical house staff (interns, residents, and specialty fellows). The term is not applied to hospitals with teaching programs for other health-care providers.

In 1989, there were 1,054 teaching community hospitals (about 19% of all community hospitals), with 393,000 beds (more than 42% of all beds in community hospitals) (AHA, 1990, Tables 6, 8). Their average size was about 370 beds, while the average size for all community hospitals was about 170 beds. They provided over 14 million admissions (almost 46% of the total to community hospitals), and on the average day cared for over 47 percent of all community-hospital patients. They provided almost one-half of all visits to community-hospital outpatient departments. Their occupancy rate was 74.6 percent, and the average length of stay was 7.5 days. Thus, teaching hospitals have an importance in the hospital system quite out of proportion to their number.

DISTRIBUTION AND RELATIVE BED SUPPLY

In 1948 there were approximately 3.4 nonfederal general-medical and surgical hospital beds per 1,000 civilian resident population (AHA, 1990, Table 1; U.S. Bureau of the Census, Table 2). By 1976, the community hospital bed to population ratio was 4.5 beds per 1,000. By 1989, the ratio had declined to 3.85. Improvements in bed distribution and increase in bed supply since World War II have been regarded as an achievement in providing access to hospitals, especially for people in rural areas. However, even the national bed-population ratio declining; given the current national community hospital occupancy rate of 66 percent, the number of hospital beds appears to be excessive. (There are regional variations. In some states, like New York, a very aggressive state health department hospital-closing policy has lead to periodic bed shortages in certain areas. Also, in certain metropolitan areas, AIDS has placed strains on the hospital system.)

The number of beds *required* for a given geographic region is a function of the number of patient days of hospital care required by the population (expressed as average daily census) and the working occupancy level deemed appropriate for the hospitals of a given area (Sattler and Bennett, p. 30), usually 90–95 percent. However, beds have not always been built in accordance with such a rational formula. Other factors include demands by the physicians for facilities for their use, local wealth and other available sources of funds, civic pride, and competition with other institutions. (Yes, even in the health-care arena, the thought "Well, if the hospital down the road has an ultraoxymegatron, we've got to have one too" obtains from time to time.)

In the past, once built, the availability of a hospital bed promoted its use (Klarman, p. 139). This relationship, "a built bed is a filled bed," was known popularly as Roemer's Law (Roemer, 1961). The filling of available beds occurred not because of overwhelming medical need in the nation; not all patients required hospitalization on medical grounds. Among the nonmedical reasons for hospital admission were patient and physician convenience, physician and hospital pecuniary gain, and the availability of hospital insurance. However, with various regulatory controls placed on hospital admissions since the mid-1970s, the occupancy rates did decline, as noted above. Unfortunately, those unfilled beds are still costly to maintain. Many hospital costs are either fixed or varied with difficulty in the face of short-term changes in utilization. These include personnel, capital construction and equipment, and utility costs. Only expenditures for food and consumable supplies do not have to be made when a bed is empty. For these reasons, it has been estimated that on a short-term basis, an empty bed costs about 70 percent as much to maintain as a filled one (Blue Cross/Blue Shield).

The only way to save money in the hospital sector is to close beds and eliminate those high fixed costs. Simply holding down admissions will not solve the problem. It saves insurance dollars in the short run but does not reduce total health expenditures by too much in the long run. Even though occupancy rates have gone down, costs have stayed up (see Chapter 7). One reason is that those empty beds are still there.

HOSPITAL STRUCTURE

Hospitals have a complex structure and a variety of administrative operating divisions. The principal ones are medical (the doctors), nursing, other diagnostic and therapeutic support, financial, personnel, hotel, and community relations. Most hospitals provide services to inpatients placed in a bed and outpatients (see Chapter 2) who come to an emergency department, an outpatient clinic, or a diagnostic or therapeutic service (such as an ambulatory surgery unit) for a procedure not requiring hospitalization, also called day hospital.

Medical Division

The medical division is organized along the lines of the several medical specialties. However, there is no universal logic to the categorization. Some are defined by the class of procedure used, some by the age or sex of their main patient group, and some by the organ or organ system that is their primary purview.

The major medical departments are:

- *Internal medicine:* diagnosis and therapy for adults, involving one or more internal organs or the skin, not requiring physical alteration of the body.
- *Surgery:* diagnosis and therapy in which physical alteration of the patient's body is usually the focus of the physician's intervention.
- *Pediatrics:* diagnosis and therapy for children, primarily using nonsurgical techniques.
- *Obstetrics/gynecology:* diagnosis and therapy focusing on the female sexual/reproductive system using both surgical and nonsurgical interventions.
- *Psychiatry:* diagnosis and therapy for people of all ages with mental and emotional problems, using counseling, pharmaceutical, and other interventions.

Other medical departments organized around organs and organ systems in which the physicians use both surgical and nonsurgical interventions include ophthalmology (eye), otolaryngology (ear, nose, and throat), urology (male sexual/reproductive system and the renal system for both males and females), orthopedics (bones and joints), and so on.

Radiology, the use of X-ray and other radiation sources, is a medical department with a primarily diagnostic function, although radiotherapy is also an important practice. In recent years, several non-X-ray, internal diagnostic techniques such as magnetic resonance imaging (MRI) have been developed. Therapeutic nuclear medicine has been separated from the diagnostic radiology in certain hospitals. Therefore, in some institutions the name of the departments whose outputs present various views of the body's interior has been changed to Diagnostic Imaging. Pathology, in medical practice, serves only a diagnostic function, both before and after treatment. Anesthesiology is principally concerned with preparing patients to be surgically operated upon without pain or discomfort during the procedure, In addition, some anesthesiologists participate in emergent or "critical-care" medicine.

Medical Staff Organization

The physician is traditionally described as a guest in the hospital and as its primary customer. The hospital is sometimes described as the doctors' workshop. Except when a physician chooses to run a hospital for profit, he has no personal responsibility to see that hospital is available to provide care for his patients. A physician is largely free to order whatever tests or treatments he deems necessary for his patient. Thus the physician is a major determinant of hospital costs, even though he bears no personal responsibility for them. He also influences the growth and expansion of the institution. Physicians' behavior is thus a major factor in the continuing rise in health-care costs.

In exchange for the privilege of admitting patients, the physician participates in governance of the medical staff and hospital, and may have to share the load for providing care in areas of the hospital for which the medical staff accepts collective responsibility, such as the emergency room or outpatient clinic. There is a wide variety of medical staff patterns of organization, which have been analyzed in great detail by Roemer and Friedman (1971).

There are many medical staff committees, responsible for overseeing the physicians' work. They include the executive committee, overall coordination and general policy setting; the joint conference committee, liaison between the medical staff and the hospital's governing board; the credentials committee, review of applications to join the medical staff; the infections-control committee, responsible for preventing infections and monitoring and correcting outbreaks of infectious disease; the pharmacy and therapeutics committee, reviews of pharmacologic agents for inclusion in the list of drugs approved for use in the hospital. There are also the tissue committee, which reviews all surgical procedures which produce "bodily tissues"; the medical records committee, responsible for certifying the completeness and clinical accuracy of the documentation of patient care; and the quality-assurance committee, which undertakes the responsibilities that its name implies.

Hospital Administration

Hospital administration keeps the institution up and running in all areas other than direct patient care. Its major responsibilities include finance, personnel, community–public relations, and the "hotel" services (maintenance, housekeeping, laundry, and dietary [cooking and delivery of meals]).

Other Health Care Divisions

The principal one is nursing (see Chapter Four). The diagnostic and therapeutic services, which may or may not be administratively attached to one of the medical departments, include laboratory (usually under the direction of the department of pathology); electrocardiography (usually a part of internal medicine); electroencephalography (part of neurology); radiotherapy technology (diagnostic imaging); pharmacy; clinical psychology; social service; inhalation therapy (often part of anesthesiology or pulmonary medicine); nutrition as therapy; physical, occupational, and speech therapy (often attached to the department of rehabilitation medicine if there is one); home care; and medical records (AHA, 1990, pp. xxi–xxiii).

HOSPITAL GOVERNANCE IN THE PRIVATE SECTOR

The typical not-for-profit hospital has a self-perpetuating board of trustees. Prominent in its membership are persons who give or raise substantial sums of money for the hospital or represent important community institutions such as major employers and banks. The "president" of the hospital is either the leader of the board of trustees, or the paid chief executive officer of the hospital. In the former case, the top paid person is usually called the executive director or executive vice president. In the latter case, the board is headed by a chairman. In theory, the board of directors sets policy, and the chief executive officer carries it out. In practice, the situation is usually as complex as in any large modern corporation.

For-profit hospitals may have a governance structure similar to that of the voluntaries, with board seats held by the owners or their representatives, or they may be run directly by the owners. All hospitals operate under the license and supervision (closer in some states than in others) of an agency of state government.

PUBLIC GENERAL HOSPITALS

The public *general* hospital (recall that there are other classes such as veterans' and mental) was defined by the Commission on Public

General Hospitals of the American Hospital Association (p. v) as "short term general and certain special hospitals excluding Federal (those operated by the Department of Defense and the Department of Veterans Affairs), psychiatric, and tuberculosis hospitals that are owned by state and local governments." As of 1989, there were 1,390 local government and 92 state government general hospitals with a total of about 170,000 beds (AHA, 1990, Table 2A). The public hospital sector is shrinking. In 1981, at the beginning of the Reagan era, there were 1,772 state and local general hospitals.

Public general hospitals provide care for many persons unable to get care elsewhere: the poor, the homeless, the street prostitute, the destitute drug addict or alcoholic, the disruptive poor psychiatric patient, the low-income elderly, and the prisoner. In certain areas, they are the only source of care for patients with special medical problems: the badly burned, the at-risk newborn, the high-risk mother, and the victim of criminal or noncriminal life-threatening trauma. While only a minority of hospitals are under public ownership, in a nation without universal health-care cost coverage, they bear an importance beyond their numbers.

THE PROBLEMS OF HOSPITALS

First, hospitals are costly places to build and maintain (see Chapter 7). Second, there is an imbalance in the hospital sector between acute and long-term care. The high costs of hospital care are exacerbated by the inadequate supply of affordable long-term-care beds for patients who have recovered from the acute phase of their illness but still need high-quality care in bed. Beyond that, there is a pressing need for appropriate housing with social and support services for the elderly who cannot live entirely on their own in ordinary housing but nevertheless do not need institutionalization of any kind (Rogatz).

The imbalance that does exist, however, by no means developed accidentally, as Freymann noted (p. 47):

> The mold from which today's health care system was cast took its shape around 1850. There were still relatively few general hospitals or health facilities of any type in Britain [our most important medical *organizational* forebear] and the fledgling United States, but the institutional organization of health care was already firmly established. Separate administration and staffing of the curative services for acute, chronic, and psychiatric illnesses became such a strong precedent that it continues even when all three components have a common source of support, as they do now in Britain.

The third major problem concerns the mode by which most physicians taking care of patients in hospitals are paid and the influence that physicians have over hospital operations. The physician makes most of the decisions on the commitment and use of hospital resources. Yet, as noted above, it is usually the patient or his insurer who pays him. Thus, he has neither a direct financial relationship to the hospital nor any responsibility for its financial health. It is as if modern school boards provided everything necessary for education except payment of the teachers, who would proceed to collect fees directly from the students. (Indeed this is the way teachers were paid before the educational reforms of the mid nineteenth century.)

Fourth, hospitals have problems with vertically organized administrative structures that are not well integrated horizontally at the service levels. In many hospitals the vertical lines of authority of the medical staff, nursing, and support-hotel services meet only in the office of the director. However, in some they never meet. This kind of separation can make it very difficult to provide integrated programs of patient care in which unitary direction is needed at the functional level to meet patient needs best (Jonas, 1973).

A fifth problem is the programmatic and sometimes philosophical isolation of many hospitals from the real health and medical problems of their communities. This does not apply solely to short-term general hospitals. For example, in many hospitals, outpatient services have a distinctly second-class status, preventive medicine is practiced to a minimal extent (although that situation is improving), home care and rehabilitation services are treated as luxuries. Community-based chronic-disease-control programs are not undertaken. Mental hospitals have little to do with community mental health. Since they want patients inside, not outside, proprietary nursing homes have not the least interest in dealing with the complications of aging in a positive way. Although change is occurring, some hospitals have resolutely turned inward, wishing that everyone would just go away and leave them to do their job as they see it: taking care of sick people in bed.

John Gordon Freyman summarized much of the situation well when he said (p. 48):

> The contrast between the history of voluntary hospitals and that of the other three fragments of the health care system [long-term, psychiatric, public health services] is striking. A common thread runs through the chronicle of the last three—entanglement with over-whelming numbers of people and with complex social, economic, and political problems. . . . Voluntary hospitals have been able to limit their involvement for almost

200 years, while the other three components sequestered the problems which were destined to become the main health concerns of the late 20th century.

SOLUTIONS

Complex problems do not have simple solutions, and there are no panaceas. But in the context of a program of universal financial entitlement to health services, an approach to hospital reform is available. We turn once again to Freymann, who developed the "mission-oriented hospital" concept (Freymann, chap. 18).

The mission-oriented hospital has two principal attributes: (1) each hospital has a mission defined and continuously modified by the specific needs of the community it services; (2) the rational planning process provides individuality and flexibility (Freymann, p. 248). Freymann (p. 247) recognized that the word 'hospital' itself presents a problem, for today it connotes a building that houses patients. I think 'hospital' could be used in a different sense to signify a dynamic complex of facilities and skilled personnel organized to provide all types of health services."

He pointed out (p. 212) that

> while general hospitals were originally only for the acutely sick, history has dictated that they become the centers about which the American health care system revolves. To consider creating new centers for the care of the well and limiting 6,000 general hospitals to their 18th century function is to fly in the face of reality. But [to meet their new functions] they must be designed [physically and programmatically] not as enclaves but as open accessible places where the scattered fragments of the health care system can at least be brought together.

The mission-oriented approach would make the hospital into a health center rather than an illness center, ending what Freymann called the "tyranny of the bed." The hospital would respond to the needs of its community in a rational, planned, dynamic manner. By definition, the acute-chronic-preventive distinctions would become relics of the past. The present administrative problems would not be automatically resolved by a mission-oriented approach; they would have to be solved to accomplish mission orientation. It demands an administrative structure that is functionally decentralized to operate integrated programs requiring staff teams at the care level, not one which has vertically organized reporting lines separating health-care providers into independent hierarchies.

A major challenge in implementing mission orientation lies in finding the personnel who can do it. To change hospitals to mission orientation will require mission-oriented physicians and other staff who can understand health and illness in populations as well as in individuals and can see patients in their socioeconomic context. But the bulk of health-sciences training takes place in our present inward-directed hospitals. How to break out of this vicious circle requires a separate discussion (Jonas, 1979). Solutions and resources are available to do so. Needed is the summoning of the political will to deal with the complex situation.

LONG-TERM CARE: THE EXAMPLE OF NURSING HOMES

There is a group of long-term institutions other than long-term hospitals, generically called nursing homes.* Their number has increased significantly since the 1930s. Formerly classified according to the level of skill involved in the care they gave, beginning in 1990, all nursing homes eligible to receive federal third-party reimbursement for the care they provide are called nursing facilities. In 1986 there were over 16,000 such institutions of 25 beds or more, with over 1.6 million beds (National Center for Health Statistics, Table 99). Occupancy rates averaged over 90 percent.

More than 75 percent of nursing homes are under for-profit ownership, with 20 percent in the voluntary sector and 5 percent owned by government agencies. Fewer than 70 percent of the beds are found in the proprietary units. More than half the financial support for nursing homes comes from public funds, much of it Medicaid since Medicare provides little long-term coverage.

Chronic problems with quality of care provoke periodic exposes and outcries for reform. But since any institutional care is expensive, the long-term solution to the long-term-care problem probably lies with improved home-care services and improved health-promotive, disease-preventive, and self-care programs for the rapidly increasing number of elderly person in the United States.

---

*Long-term care deserves a much more complete discussion than we have room for in this book. Much of this short section is based on Hila Richardson, "Long Term Care," chap. 8 in *Health Care Delivery in the United States*, 4th ed., ed. A. Kovner, (New York: Springer Publishing, 1990). The reader is referred to this excellent chapter for more detail on nursing homes in particular and long-term care in general.

REFERENCES

AHA, American Hospital Association. *Hospital Statistics, 1979*. Chicago: 1979.

AHA, American Hospital Association. *Hospital Statistics 1990–91*, Chicago: 1990.

Blue Cross/Blue Shield of Greater New York. "Just How Much Hospital Capacity Does This City Need?" *New York Times*, August 24, 1976.

Commission on Public General Hospitals. *The Future of the Public General Hospital*. Chicago: Hospital Research and Educational Trust, 1978.

Freymann, J. G. *The American Health Care System: Its Genesis and Trajectory*. New York: Medcom Press, 1974.

Jonas, S. "Some Thoughts on Primary Care: Problems in Implementation." *International Journal of Health Services, 3*, 177, 1973.

Jonas, S. *Medical Mystery: The Training of Doctors in the United States*. New York: W. W. Norton, 1979.

Klarman, H. E., *The Economics of Health*, New York: Columbia University Press, 1965.

Knowles, J. "The Hospital." In S. J. Williams, ed., *Issues in Health Services*. New York: Wiley, 1980.

MacEachern, M. T. *Hospital Organization and Management*. Berwyn, IL: Physician's Record, 1962.

NCHS, National Center for Health Statistics. *Health: United States, 1989*. Hyattsville, MD: DHHS Pub. No. (PHS) 90-1232, 1990.

Roemer, M.I. "Bed Supply and Hospital Utilization: A Natural Experiment." *Hospitals, J.A.H.A.*, November 1961.

Roemer, M.I., Friedman, J. W. *Doctors in Hospitals*. Baltimore: Johns Hopkins University Press, 1971.

Rogatz, P. M. "Directions of Health System for the New Decade." *Hospitals*, January 1, 1980, p. 67.

Rosenberg, C. E. "The Origins of the American Hospital System." *Bulletin of the New York Academy of Medicine, 55*, 10, 1979.

Sattler, F. L., Bennett, M. D. *A Statistical Profile of Short-Term Hospitals in the United States as of 1973*. Minneapolis: Interstudy, 1975.

Stern, B. J. *Medical Services by Government*. New York: Commonwealth Fund, 1946.

Stevens, R. *American Medicine and the Public Interest*. New Haven, CT: Yale University Press, 1971.

U.S. Bureau of the Census. *Statistical Abstract of the United States, 1990*. Washington, DC: 1979.

Chapter 4

Personnel

OVERVIEW

In 1988 almost 8.8 million people, about 8 percent of all persons employed, were working in the health-care industry.* About half of them worked in hospitals, 17 percent in nursing and personal-care facilities, and 11 percent in physicians' offices. Among the health-care professionals, there were about 1,627,000 active registered nurses, 538,000 physicians, 156,000 pharmacists, 140,000 dentists, 46,000 veterinarians, 26,000 optometrists, and 11,000 podiatrists, and in the community hospitals (see Chapter 3) alone, close to 35,000 dieticians, about 32,000 physical therapists, and over 17,000 social workers. In the community hospitals there were also about 760,000 licensed practical nurses, more than 145,000 laboratory personnel, close to 100,000 radiologic service personnel, and about 55,000 respiratory therapists and technicians.

The ratio of other health personnel to physicians reflects the complexity of the U.S. health-care system. In 1987, there were about 470,000 physicians in active practice. There were almost 18 other health-care workers for each doctor. This compares with about 3 other health-care workers per doctor in 1920 (Donabedian et al.). Most of these other personnel have skills learned through special training. Only about one-fifth are nonspecific clerical, custodial, or similar personnel.

Altogether, the U.S. Department of Labor has identified about 700 categories of skilled health occupations. Under the laws of most states, only physicians (allopathic, M.D., and osteopathic, D.O.), den-

---

*Except as otherwise noted, the data used in this chapter are taken from *Health United States, 1989*, National Center for Health Statistics, Hyattsville, MD: DHHS Pub. No. (PHS) 90-1232, 1990, pp. 3–4, Tables 83–92 (abbreviated NCHS).

tists, and a few other types of practitioner may serve patients directly without the authorization of a health professional licensed for independent practice. Among the other independent health professions are chiropractic, optometry, podiatry, psychotherapy, and in some states, midwifery and phsycial therapy. For the most part, nurses work on the orders of physicians, although in certain circumstances in certain states, some nurses practice independently.

Other types of health-care providers, working on the orders and under at least the general supervision of physicians, include clinical laboratory, X-ray, electrocardiographic, and other specialized technicians such as those who operate kidney dialysis machines. In rehabilitation service there are physical, occupational, and speech therapists. For dental care there are dental hygienists, dental technicians, and dental assistants. Nutritionists and dietitians, statisticians and statistical clerks, medical record librarians and information system specialists, cardiorespiratory therapists, audiologists, and plaster cast technicians perform other special tasks.

Many of these occupations developed out of the nursing profession. In countries less developed than the United States, the work of the laboratory technician, physical therapist, or dietitian may at present be done by the nurse. But in the United States the work is now done by specialists. Further, the diversification and specialization in medicine that occurred as medical science and technology advanced and became more complex took place in the nursing profession too. Consider, for example, the development of the operating-room nurse, the intensive-care nurse, and the nurse anesthetist. In the next two sections, we consider the two largest health professions, medicine and nursing, in more detail.

PHYSICIANS

Basic Data

According to the Medical Practice Act of New York State (Article 131, Para. 6521, of the State Education Law) (USNY, 1989, p. 27), medical practice is "diagnosing, treating, operating or prescribing for any human disease, pain, injury, deformity or physical condition." To qualify for a medical license in New York State, one must (USNY, pp. 27, 36) hold an M.D. or D.O. degree or its equivalent from a school meeting the State Education Department's requirements, have certain postgraduate practice experience, pass a specified exam, be a citizen or resident alien, be of "good moral character," and pay a fee. (All states have similar requirements.)

As of 1987, about 89 percent of the 585,000 presently or formerly licensed U.S. physicians were in active practice (NCHS, Table 86).* About 21 percent of the 521,000 active physicians received their medical training outside the United States and Canada. Almost 22,000 of the active physicians were in federal government service, most of them in the armed forces or the U.S. Public Health Service. More than three-quarters of the federal physicians worked in patient-care services.

About 453,000 (90%) of all nonfederal physicians worked in patient care. Of those, about 75 percent were in office-based practice, more than 17 percent were house staff (interns and residents in training), and almost 8 percent were full-time hospital-based practitioners (NCHS, Table 86). About 114,000 physicians were in group practice, both private and prepaid (AMA) (see Chapter 2). The more than 46,000 nonfederal professionally active physicians who were not in patient care worked in administration, medical education, research, state and local health services, the pharmaceutical industry, and the like. The largest physician specialties were general and family practice and internal medicine, each with about 55,000; obstetrics and gynecology, with more than 24,000; and general surgery and pediatrics, both with over 23,000.

In 1987, the overall physician-to-population ratio was 22.6 per 10,000 (NCHS, Table 85). This is up from a post–World War II low in 1960 of 14 per 10,000. Of the geographic regions, New England reported the highest ratio, 27.7 per 10,000, while the East South Central (Kentucky, Tennessee, Alabama, and Mississippi) reported the lowest, 15.9. By state, the ratio ranged from a low of 7.7 in South Dakota to a high of 23.8 in California. While there are no known differences in health status that vary consistently with physician-population ratios, utilization of health services in generally higher in those areas that have more physicians (Eisenberg, pp. 15–17; Leape et al.; Wennberg). Among the factors influencing the amount of work physicians do are income goals, desired practice style, personal characteristics, practice setting, and standards established by clinical leadership (Eisenberg, chap. 2).

---

*Please note that there are some slight, unexplained, inconsistencies between the several tables reporting physician supply in *Health:United States, 1989.*

Private Medical Practice

The primary mode of organization in the United States (and indeed of most other health-care providers who are licensed to practice independently) is private practice. The private practitioner contracts directly with patients (although almost never in writing) to provide a set of services in return for a fee. This arrangement is called the fee-for-service system. A combination of the licensing laws of the state in which he is located, the requirements of his malpractice insurer, and the stipulations of the hospital to which he admits patients if he is a hospital staff member, regulate what the physician in private practice may do to and for patients.

In 1989 about 75 percent of all physicians who were in active practice, including hospital-based physicians but excluding house staff, were in private practice (Gillis & Wilke). While the trend slowed to a standstill in the late 1980s, the proportion of physicians working on salary has been increasing, especially for younger physicians. Among the reasons are the attractiveness of a regular salary and a compreshensive fringe-benefit package; the provision of malpractice insurance by the employer; regular hours and regular nights and weekends schedules; the difficulty of entering into private practice in many desirable living areas, many of which are already over-doctored; the high costs of starting private practice, a special burden to so many of today's new physicians who start professional life with a large debt accumulated in the course of their medical education.

Patterns of Practice

An important feature of the U.S. private-practice sector is that most physicians see patients on an ambulatory basis in their offices and as hospital inpatients. (A small percentage of doctors do not have hospital appointments. How many is not known. Most are probably in urban areas.) In most other countries, physicians see ambulatory patients only or work full-time in hospitals. The unusual American arrangement offers some significant advantages to the patient. For the many conditions for which one physician is technically competent to provide both ambulatory and inpatient care, there is continuity of care. In many cases requiring surgery, the nonsurgical referring physician will participate in the pre- and postoperative phases in the hospital.

Medical Specialization

Specialization is a prominent feature of American medical practice.* The explosion of biomedical knowledge and technology that began early in this century has made it ever more difficult for a physician to master more than one small piece of what biomedical science and practice can do. (The specialties of family medicine, primary-care pediatrics, and primary-care internal medicine still demand a very broad range of knowledge and competencies. In a way, however, most specialization makes the practice of medicine easier for the physician by focusing on a relatively narrow range of knowledge and skill, even though they may be required in great depth.) The way American specialization has developed, there is always more money to be made in the specialties. And finally, there has never been a health-personnel planning policy in this country.

Specialization has its advantages for patients. Specialists develop a high degree of knowledge and skill in dealing with their areas of expertise. But it also has its disadvantages. Specialists tend to concentrate on one organ or organ system. The patient's well-being may suffer if there is no professional who can (1) see her as a whole person; (2) put together into one clinical picture a variety of complaints arising from different organ systems; (3) guide her through an intelligent utilization of the knowledge of several specialists; and (4) set up an organized means for communication among specialists. This argument is not against specialization per se; the vast expansion of medical knowledge requires such specialization, at least for a certain proportion of the profession. It is for a more rational approach to the organization of specialists and a significant improvement in the provision of primary-care physician services (Colwill; Geyman; Relman; White).

Patients, particularly those who use the private sector and thus can pick their own points of entry, face a sometimes bewildering array of

---

*A particularly erudite and detailed history of the development of specialization in American medical practice is presented by Rosemary Stevens in her still timely history *American Medicine and the Public Interest* (New Haven, CN: Yale University Press, 1971).

physicians to choose from. Many private-sector patients create what might be called a "group practice in the mind." It includes, perhaps, "my" internist, "my" psychiatrist, "my" neurologist, "my" allergist, "my" surgeon, "my" obstetrician-gynecologist, and so on. (Hopefully, it does not include "my" pathologist.)

This means that when a patient notices a new symptom (something felt or experienced) or a new sign (something noticed objectively by the patient or other observer), it is the patient, usually an untrained observer, who evaluates its meaning and picks an entry point in the spectrum of specialists. Unfortunately for many patients, few members of the "group practice in the mind" know each other; thus, communication among them is often poor. Poor communication among physican specialists can well lead to a less than optimum outcome for the patient.

Medical Education

As of July 1990, there were 125 fully accredited medical schools offering the M.D. degree and 16 offering the D.O. degree in the United States.* M.D. medical schools in the United States and Canada are accredited by a voluntary agency called the Liaison Committee on Medical Education. It is composed of representatives from the American Medical Association (AMA) and the Association of American Medical Colleges (AAMC) and their Canadian counterparts. Osteopathic (D.O.) medical schools, found only in the United States, are accredited by the American Osteopathic Association.

All but a few medical schools are attached to a university. The medical school is a separate college, sometimes loosely linked with other health professional schools in a "health sciences center." About half the medical schools are sponsored by state governments as part of state public universities, and half are under private auspices. All the schools, however, have received substantial financial support from the federal government for many years.

Entry to U.S. medical schools usually requires a university bachelor's degree (requiring four years of study). The standard medical-school program, called undergraduate medical education, lasts another four years. Although there have been some changes in recent years, most schools employ a standard curriculum: two years of

*The data on medical education are drawn from "Medical Education in the United States, 1989–90," American Medical Association, *Journal of the American Medical Association, 264,* 791, 1990.

didactic basic science study followed by two years of clinical study with patients.

In the United States, medical licensure is granted by the states. The first requirement is graduation from an accredited medical school. In addition, the candidate must undertake at least one year of additional training in a hospital (the "internship" or "postGraduate year [PGY] one") and pass the U.S. Medical Licensure Examination (this exam was created in 1990 by merger of the old National Board of Medical Examiners and Federation of State Medical Boards exams). In practice, in the 1990s, few medical-school graduates enter practice before completing at least three more years of training in what is called a residency.

Admission to medical schools is selective. In 1990, there were about 27,000 applicants, of whom about 17,000 found places. The ratio of applicants to places, now 1.6, has been falling steady since it reached a high of 2.8 in 1973–1975. The proportion of women in medical school has been increasing steadily since the early 1970s. In 1990, women accounted for 39 percent of the number of applicants, 38 percent of the entering class, and one-third of the graduating class that entered four years before.

The record for admissions for Afro-Americans does not match that for women (NCHS, Table 92). Although the medical schools have made some efforts since the 1970s to increase Afro-American admissions, the percentage has remained unchanged, at about 6, and 16 percent of all Afro-American medical students attend one of the three primarily Afro-American medical schools. At the same time, Hispanic admissions have increased moderately, Native-American admissions have remained low (less than 0.5 percent), and Asian-American admissions have quadrupled.

The ratio of full-time faculty to students is very low, less than 1.2. This is one of the reasons medical education is so expensive. In 1989–1990, the medical schools collectively spent close to $17 billion to educate only 140,000 medical students, basic-science graduate students, and hospital residents, more than $120,000 each per year. Of course, included in that figure are the salaries and stipends for residents and graduate students. And medical schools do much else besides train physicians. Over 19 percent of their budgets are spent on research, about 23 percent on health and community service. But that per-student cost is high. And while tuition and fees account for only 4.5 percent of total medical-school expenditures, it is not unusual for a student to graduate $100,000 in debt for undergraduate and medical education.

NURSING

The American Nurses Association (ANA, 1981) has defined nursing*
as:

> assessment, diagnosis, planning, intervention, and evaluation in the pro-
> motion and maintenance of health; the casefinding and management of
> illness, injury, or infirmity; the restoration of optimum function; or the
> achievement of a dignified death. Nursing practice includes but is not
> limited to administration, teaching, counseling, supervision, delegation,
> and evaluation of practice and execution of the medical regimen, includ-
> ing the administration of medications and treatments prescribed by any
> person authorized by state law to prescribe.

According to the Nursing Practice Act of New York State (Article
139, Para. 6902 of the State Education Law) (USNY, 1990, p. 27),

> The practice of the profession of nursing as a registered professional
> nurse is defined as diagnosing and treating human responses to actual or
> potential health problems through such services as casefinding, health
> teaching, health counseling, and provision of care supportive to or re-
> storative of life and well-being, and executing medical regimens pre-
> scribed by a licensed or otherwise legally authorized physician or den-
> tist. A nursing regimen shall be consistent with and not vary any existing
> medical regimen.

Further, the act states (Para. 6901) (USNY, p. 27):

> "Diagnosing" in the context of nursing practice means that identification
> of and discrimination between physical and psychosocial signs and
> symptoms essential to effective execution and management of the nurs-
> ing regimen. "Treating" means selection and performance of those
> therapeutic measures essential to the effective execution and manage-
> ment of the nursing regimen, and execution of any prescribed medical
> regimen. "Human responses" means those signs, symptoms and pro-
> cesses which denote the individual's interaction with an actual or poten-
> tial health problem.

According to the ANA, the human responses concerning nurses
include self-care limitations; impaired functioning in areas ranging
from rest and sleep to nutrition and sexuality; pain and discomfort;

---

*For more details on nursing, see chapter 5, "Nursing," by Christine Kovner, in *Health
Care Delivery in the United States*, 4th ed., ed. Anthony Kovner (New York: Springer
Publishing, 1990).

emotional difficulties; deficiencies in personal decision making from a variety of causes; and stress related to significant life events—birth, death, divorce, serious disability (ANA, 1980, p. 10). Nurturing is the human characteristic basic to all nursing functions. (Note that the definition of nursing is much more detailed than that of medicine [see above]).

Properly made, nursing diagnoses are measurable and reproducible. Such diagnoses are defined in terms of human behaviors and problems for which there are nursing interventions, as distinct from medical interventions. Each diagnosis is described by etiology, defining characteristics, and the expectations for nursing interventions (Kim, McFarland, & McLane).

Nursing has changed from an earlier intuitive practice to a scientifically defined and defensible one. This change provides a new level of nurse autonomy and accountability. Identifiable and measurable services pave the way for different types of payment for nursing and create the opportunity for new working environments. Problems covered by nursing diagnoses are frequently those that also extend hospital stay.

The practice of nursing long had to overcome social objections to a female's intimate access to the bodies of strangers of both sexes. Traditionally, such access was permissible only for healers and servants. Healing implied special learning, tools, and secret knowledge. In the past, many observers viewed the commonly visible clinical skills of nursing as those of the parent, and thus menial, requiring mainly common sense. The skills were regarded as those of untrained servants or dedicated volunteers.

The basic fallacy of the latter viewpoint has been stated repeatedly for over a century (although that does not stop some from still holding to it). In 1854 Florence Nightingale traveled to the Crimea in response to a British mandate to improve hospital care during the Crimean War. Her first problem was finding qualified nurses. Her second problem was to convince the military physicians that the care she and her nurses proposed to provide would not spoil the soldiers by "coddling the brutes." Third, she had to show that she had special skills and knowledge that could benefit the war effort.

Her nursing reforms eventually reduced hosptial mortality from 60 percent to little more than 1 percent. This did not prevent repeated attempts to undermine the program and eliminate the nurses. In the U.S. Army, soldiers in the Spanish-American War and World War I suffered while nurses struggled for the right to provide qualified nursing care. It was not until 1944 that nurses in the military forces were granted temporary status as officers. Only in 1947 did Congress establish permanent Army and Navy Nurse corps (Kalisch & Kalisch).

The heterogeneity of the U.S. health-care system has created a need for nurses in many types of service. About half of registered nurses work in hospitals, the balance primarily in nursing homes for the chronically ill, public health agencies, schools, industrial clinics, nursing education, private medical or dental offices, and private-duty positions. The employment turnover among registered nurses is high. After a few years of service, many leave nursing for other types of employment.

Categories of Nurses and Nursing Education

There are three major groups of nurses: the registered nurse (RN), the licensed practical nurse (LPN), and nurse's aides, orderlies, attendants, home health aides, and so on. The RNs have the higest level of education, the most responsibility under the states' nurse-practice acts, and the most authority. Generally, LPNs and aides function under the supervision of an RN.

Nursing is the largest health professional group. In 1988, there were about 1,627,000 active registered nurses in the United States. About 1 million of them had associate degrees or hospital-based nursing-school diplomas, more than 465,000 had baccalaureate degrees, and over 100,000 had graduate degrees. The registered nurse–population ratio was about 665 per 100,000.

Nursing is a multitiered profession. One cannot assume from the term *nurse* alone a given level of competence. "Registration" in nursing was originally a voluntary function of the nursing profession. It now means state licensure, at a significantly higher level of responsibility and authority than that accorded to the licensed practical nurse. The term *registered nurse* (RN) means that one is licensed by the state to practice professional nursing.

To be a registered nurse requires a high school diploma and a diploma from a hospital-based program, a bachelor of science in nursing (B.S.N.) from a college or university, or, since 1952, associate degree in nursing (A.D.N.) from a two-year college program. Graduate education for registered nurses is found in both college and university master's and doctoral programs. Increasingly, these advanced practitioners are also certified by governmental and/or professional bodies.

Licensed practical nurses (LPNs), called licensed vocational nurses (LVNs) in two states, may or may not have completed high school before entering a 12- to 18-month training program. LPN programs are operated by a variety of institutions, including adult schools, junior colleges, and technical schools. Like RNs, LPNs must pass a state-supervised examination to become licensed, but their work requires a significantly lower level of skill and knowledge. The education of the aides group is highly variable. Some take a formal educational program. For others, the training is primarily on the job.

In the work setting, the mix of RNs, LPN/LVNs, aides, orderlies, and so on is determined by the nature of care provided, government regulation, budget, and available manpower. Financial incentives have been provided in some state legislation to encourage facilities such as nursing homes to employ better-qualified nursing staff.

Nursing Education History

Just as nursing is multitiered, so historically has been the educational preparation for nursing practice. In the United States, formal training for nursing was first introduced in 1873 (Kalisch & Kalisch). It was provided by hospitals, which offered their graduates a diploma. By 1910, many hospitals had discovered that their nursing schools provided a convenient source of low-cost labor and came to depend on their schools for that purpose. Often there was little concern for the quality of the student's education. Lectures, when they were not canceled, were held after long hours of work. Libraries and laboratories, if they existed at all, were inadequate. Direct supervision of the younger student's clinical experience depended heavily on senior students. Some hospitals hired out students for private-duty nursing in patients' homes to increase hospital earnings.

Concern about the poor quality of these programs eventually led to a national study, the *Goldmark Report*, published in 1923. This report revealed that while there were some good schools, the average hospital was not equipped to provide more than a casual education poorly related to the students' clinical experience. The health of students was being damaged by the conditions under which they lived, worked, and studied. While the report recognized the key role of hospitals in the clinical training of nurses, it strongly recommended that the education process be under the control of educational institutions. Colleges and universities were better equipped to provide the necessary libraries, laboratories, classrooms, and instructors in the basic sciences required for professional education.

However, it was not until the national emergency of World War II that significant reforms were undertaken. One must keep in mind that women achieved the right to vote only in 1920. The education of women was not previously a high priority. In 1942, Congress passed legislation authorizing the Cadet Nurse Corps. Nursing leaders could at last develop and enforce standards for the accreditation of school facilities, faculties, and curricula. The federal government provided funds to help schools meet these standards. The magnitude of the task was shown in the *Brown Report* of 1948. Some 97 percent of nursing schools were still under hospital control. Even if a change to higher-education-based nurse education was to be undertaken, few nurses were prepared academically to hold faculty positions in colleges and universities.

Much of the opposition to nurse education in institutions of higher learning has come from the nursing profession itself. Only in the early 1980s was the consensus reached by all of the major national nursing organizations that nursing education belonged in an academic setting. It was finally agreed that entry into practice at the professional level would require the baccalaureate degree; at the technical level, the associate degree. By 1990, the majority of registered nurses in the United States received their training in these academic courses, lasting two years. They acquired their practical experience principally after becoming employed. As in several other professions in this country, nursing leadership sought continuous upgrading, and university-based programs developed, turning out nurses with bachelor's degrees.

Formal preparation and licensure for practical nurses had become widespread in the early 1950s during a nursing shortage following World War II. In 1984, LPN programs nationally became committed to extending their training to 18 months. They would then become the technical nurses envisioned as the second category of nurses by the major registered nursing organizations.

Nurses in Expanded Roles

Nurses have traditionally expanded their practice through on-the-job training. Only later was such preparation formalized in an educational program. Thus, the first public health nurses, who appeared during World War I; the first maternal and child nurses, who came on the scene in the early 1920s; the first nurse anesthetists, nurse midwives, clinical nurse specialists, and nurse practitioners were all prepared outside the formal educational system.

In each instance, the initial informal efforts were followed by the establishment of standards, formal curricula in approved programs, and more recently, the preparation for advanced levels through master's programs in universities. Usually, the first formal programs for expanded nursing work were federally funded in an attempt to meet some major public-health problem facing the country. Often these programs initially required waivers of state laws restricting nurse practice because they exposed what before had been covert nursing practice. The principles and content of nursing had not changed, but the public recognition of its scope had.

The acceptance of nursing's role in practice has led to changes in nurse-practice laws across the country. These changes have led to challenges in the courts from threatened members of other health professions. However, no differences have been demonstrated between the quality of care provided by qualified nurses and that provided by physicians (Record et al.). There is good evidence that properly prepared nurses in advanced practice can provide much of normal pregnancy care and delivery, primary ambulatory care, and routine anesthesia at least as well as physicians. Physician control over access to care, through licensure and reimbursement for services, is therefore being challenged as an economic issue and against the public interest (Aiken, 1982). The ultimate battle may be over restraint of trade.

In 1988, New York State, following the lead of some other states, formalized the nurse-practitioner role in its education law (USNY, para. 6902 [3]):

> The practice of registered professional nursing by a nurse practitioner . . . may include the diagnosis of illness and physical conditions and the performance of therapeutic and corrective measures . . . in collaboration with a licensed physician . . . provided such services are performed in accordance with a written practice agreement and written practice guidelines. The written practice agreement shall include explicit provisions for the resolution of any disagreement between the collaborating physician and the nurse practitioner regarding . . . diagnosis or treatment . . . within the scope of practice of both. To the extent the practice agreement does not so provide, then the collaborating physician's diagnosis or treatment shall prevail.

This sort of legislation opens the door for truly expanded nurse practice. That can be a boon to patients, especially in such areas as primary care. To the extent that it draws nurses from traditional roles, especially in the hospital, it may well be aggravating the nursing shortage.

The Nursing Shortage

Nursing shortages have appeared periodically in the United States. The one of the early 1950s, which lead to the formalization of licensed practical nurse training and requirements, was mentioned above. Entering the 1990s, another one was upon us (Aiken & Mullinix; ANA, 1990; Secretary's Commission on Nursing). In 1990, the U.S. Department of Health and Human Services (USDHHS) estimated the nursing shortage to be about 200,000 *(Premier Focus)*. It predicted shortages of about 350,000 in the year 2000, 520,000 in 2010, and 875,000 in 2020. In 1988 the RN vacancy rate in hospitals was over 11 percent. In the face of this situation, nursing school enrollments are actually declining, and minority recruitment is lagging. Curious is the fact that if half the approximately 400,000 RNs not working in nursing (ANA, 1990) were doing so, there would be no nursing shortage.

Authorities on the subject have cited many reasons to account for this state of affairs, among them low salaries (the average starting salary for a staff nurse in 1988 was $25,000); limited chances for significant increases in pay over the life of a career (the average maximum salary for a *head* nurse in 1988 was $45,000); working conditions (high-tech work creates much stress; shift work is a serious problem); poor professional image; and widening career opportunities for women (for those starting out in life and RNs). But the doctor-nurse relationship is key (Stein et al.). As Aiken and Mullinix point out, "Much of the dissatisfaction of nurses with hospital practice is related to the absence of satisfying professional relationships with physicians."

What to do? Proposed solutions abound. One set focuses on establishing some new category of sub-RN nursing staff to take up the slack. This appears to have much in common with the LPN strategy of the 1950s. The American Medical Association proposed the creation of the "registered care technician" (RCT) (Stein, et al.). The RCT would be trained in the hospital (like the original hospital-based-diploma nurse) and be primarily responsible for carrying out the doctor's orders in such matters as medications, test ordering, and discharge arrangements (like the original hospital-based-diploma nurse). (Apparently those newfangled degreed nurses insist on questioning doctors' orders with increasing frequency, creating a problem for the doctors beyond the simple nursing shortage.) The ANA comments that the AMA proposal "was designed to return to bedside nursing 'to a devalued, low-paying, subservient field of practice' " (Stein et al.).

The Center for Nursing of the American Hospital Association made a proposal for an occupation called the "nurse extender" (NE) *(American Hospital News*, December 3, 1990). Unlike the AMA's RCT, the NE reports to the nurse, not the doctor. The NE is responsible for carrying out the many nursing tasks for which the RN education is not required (again, shades of the LPN). These include dealing with patient hygiene, nutritional, and mobility needs, and clerical, supply-stocking, and patient-transport functions. However, among those tasks is *not* simply carrying out doctors' orders while bypassing the RN on the hospital floor.

The RCT idea is apparently dead in the water. NEs are coming on line all over the country, even though they are apparently low-paid and "subservient" (characteristics of the proposed RCT about which the ANA complained). But note that the subservience of the NE, if it exists, is to nurses, not doctors. The power relationships in the hospitals may be starting to change, after all.

The other set of proposed solutions focuses on making registered nursing itself more attractive (Aiken & Mullinix; Helmer & McKnight; Neylan). First among them is raising the pay. However, in the early 1990s, hospitals were facing significant financial squeezes. At the federal level, there were the massive Medicare cuts over five years of the 1990 Deficit Reduction Act (*American Hospital News*, November 12, 1990). At the state level, government after government faced tax and spending crises. These were secondary to the Reagan federal cuts of the 1980s and the concurrent slashing of aid to the states under the so-called New Federalism (Tolchin). The latter transferred authority from the federal government to the states and cut federal funds for many national domestic programs the Reagan administration did not like. In this climate, significant pay raises for RNs were unlikely.

Among other steps for which there was more hope of implementation were more-creative solutions to the nights-and-weekends-shifts problem; giving nurses more control over their work; expanding nurse participation in hospital decision making; improving continuing professional education; restructuring the work of the nurse (part of which is the further extension of the nurse extender concept); developing better career ladders for nurses (although that would cost money).

At the center of it all remains the need to change the rules of the "doctor-nurse game" further (Stein et al.). After all, not all of those 400,000 RNs who in 1990 were not nursing chose to leave the profession simply because they were burned out, too old, having children, wanted to stay home, or thought some other line of work would be more fun. For some of them certainly, the problem (Aiken and Muilinix) was that "much of the dissatisfaction of nurses with hospital practice is related to the absence of satisfying professional relationships with physicians."

THE PHYSICIAN ASSISTANT

The profession of physician assistant (PA) has developed in the United States since the Vietnam War (1965–1973).* It has become complex and multifaceted (Schafft & Cawley). The PA's role (Schafft & Cawley, p. 6) is to:

• Approach a patient of any age group in any setting to elicit a detailed and accurate history, perform an appropriate physical examination, delineate problems, and record and present patient data.
• Analyze health status data obtained via interview, examination, and laboratory diagnostic studies and delineate health care problems in consultation with the physician.
• Formulate, implement, and monitor an individualized treatment and/ or management plan for a patient in consultation with the physician.
• Instruct and counsel patients regarding compliance with the prescribed therapeutic regimen, normal growth and development, family planning, emotional problems of daily living, and health maintenance.
• Perform routine procedures essential to managing simple conditions produced by infection or trauma, assist in the management of more complex illness and injury, and initiate evaluations and therapeutic procedures in response to life-threatening situations.

From the creation of the PA profession (which occurred just before the Vietnam War but received a big boost from all the returning medics from it), it was conceived as an "extension" of the physician. It was not to be a separate profession like nursing. In each state, PA licensure is provided for under the medical-practice act. And although the sex balance has changed over the years, in the beginning the PA profession was predominately male. For these two reasons, many of the male-chauvinist–power issues that cloud the relationship between physicians and nurses did not appear.

There are more than 50 PA training programs. Most of them are in medical schools or schools of the allied health professions in four-year colleges. In 1986 there were an estimated 18,000 PA's in the United States. While in the early days most PA's were going into primary care, in the 1980s specialization became common. PA's work for individual physicians and in corporate settings. Like nurse prac-

---

*At the 1972 annual meeting of the American Public Health Association there was a panel presentation on new health-care developments in Canada that included a discussion of the nurse practitioner. This author asked if there were PA programs in Canada. The speaker replied: "We don't need to have PA programs. We have had no Vietnam War with the large number of returning medics to use and provide for. We need only nurse practitioner programs."

titioners, PA's provide care that is comparable in quality to that provided by physicians seeing the same kinds of patients.

HEALTH PERSONNEL FOR PRIMARY CARE

As noted in Chapter 2, by sheer volume, primary health-care services are primary. In the late 1960s, a task list for the ideal primary-care system was developed that is still valid (Committee on Medical Schools, p. 753):

1. Assessment of total patient needs before these are categorized by specialty.
2. Elaboration of a plan for meeting those needs in the order of their importance.
3. Determination of who shall meet the defined needs—physicians (generalist or specialist); nonphysician members of the health care team; or social agencies.
4. Follow-up to see that needs are met.
5. Provision of such care in a continuous, coordinated and comprehensive manner.
6. Attention at each step . . . to the personal, social and family dimensions of the patient's problem.
7. The provision of health maintenance and disease prevention at the same level of importance as the provision of cure and rehabilitation.

This description of functions shows that physician primary care is not simply a collection of services but above all a state of mind (Committee on Medical Schools, p. 754):

The primary-care physician must be capable of establishing a profile of the total needs of the patient and his family. This evaluation should include social, economic, and psychological details as well as the more strictly "medical" aspects. He must know what resources are available for meeting those needs. He should then define a plan of care, deciding which parts are to be carried out by himself and which by others. The plan should have a long-range dimension. It should be understandable to the patient and his family, and it should include a follow-up on whether indicated measures have been undertaken and whether they have been effective.

In the 1990s, of course, the task-list and state-of-mind requirements apply to primary-care nurse practitioners and physician assistants as well as primary-care physicians. The important questions in primary care are (Schwenk & Wooley):

- Who are the "appropriately trained health professionals?"
- What are their attitudes and approach to health care and the patient?
- What is their training?

One might think that physician primary care would be provided solely by family practitioners, the successors to the old-time general practitioner (GP). (The GP was often a medical-school graduate who took no more than a one-year internship and then went into practice. There are few of them left.) Family practitioners usually take a three-year residency that includes general adult medicine, general pediatrics, routine obstetrics, minor surgery, and office psychiatry. They are prepared to deliver primary-care services to entire families. This new specialty has grown rapidly since its inception in 1969. By 1987, there were over 55,000 family (and general) practitioners in office-based practice.

General pediatricians and specialists in general internal medicine (i.e., members of these broad specialties who have not further subspecialized in such areas as cardiology or neurology) are also well prepared, but they are trained to care only for children or only for adults. One of the unresolved battles in the continuing evolution of primary care is among those who favor the family practitioner as the basic primary-care doctor, those who favor the separate treatment of adults and children by internists and pediatricians, and those who favor family care by internist-pediatrician teams (Colwill; Geyman; Relman).

Nurse practitioners and physicians assistants trained in family, general adult, or general pediatric care have become significant providers of primary care. Whether they should function as "physician extenders" or as independent primary-care practitioners remains an unresolved debate (Record et al.). In some parts of the country, nurse practitioners have begun to set up independent private practices.

The primary-care role of the obstetrician-gynecologist is also unclear. When family practitioners skilled in routine obstetrics provide primary care, the obstetrician-gynecologist functions in a secondary, consultative role. A third model is familiar to any young woman whose only ongoing relationship with a doctor is with the obstetrician-gynecologist she sees for contraceptive services and pregnancy care. As a healthy young adult, she will have few nonobstetrical medical problems and will naturally bring these to the only doctor she knows. Recognizing this relationship of de facto primary care, the American Medical Association includes obstetricians in its definition of primary-care physicians. It is likely that the debate over who should be doing what to whom in primary care will continue for many years to come.

HEALTH PERSONNEL IN VARIOUS SETTINGS

There are many settings in which health services are provided and many categories of health workers who provide them. In this section, we present a few examples of each.

Mental Health Centers

The personnel requirements of facilities for ambulatory mental health services include psychologists, psychiatric social workers and nurses, carefully chosen receptionists, and psychiatrists. Community outreach workers are a new type of personnel trained in recent years by ambulatory-care programs, general and mental. These are typically (but not always) young women from the service area who may have no background in the health field but understand local attitudes. After brief training, they visit families and encourage them to make use of the health services being offered.

School Health Services

Most often, the key health person is a part-time or full-time school nurse, usually engaged by the local education authorities but sometimes assigned by the public health agency. School physicians, who examine children to detect physical or mental disorders, are principally part-time private practitioners; in some large school districts, such as New York or Los Angeles, they may be full-time salaried doctors.

Since childhood problems that may retard learning are naturally of greatest concern in school systems, other specialists are often employed. There may be psychologists for identifying mental and emotional difficulties and occasionally medical social workers and special-education teachers. For discovery of hearing defects (which may often be overlooked), audiologists are sometimes engaged. Dental hygienists may also work in school systems to inspect teeth and educate children about sound dental habits.

Local Health Department Centers

Public-health nurses are the mainstay of the clinics that focus on preventive services in addition to part-time physicians who are otherwise mainly in private practice. Other personnel in public-health clinics include health educators, nutritionists or dietitians, sexually transmitted disease (STD) investigators, and various clerks. Beyond the personnel working in various clinics, public health agencies require sanitarians (to monitor environmental conditions), statisticians, community-health educators with specialized skills, and sometimes persons trained specifically in family planning.

Occupational Health

Companies that have especially hazardous workplaces may employ industrial hygienists on a full- or part-time basis. These are personnel with special knowledge of factory or mining problems and methods by which they may be controlled. Industrial nurses and physicans can be better prepared for their work through special training programs. The federal Occupational Safety and Health Act of 1970 was a landmark in this field, even though there have been serious limitations in the implementation of its regulations.

Pharmacies

In some countries, where pharmacies are devoted almost exclusively to the sale of medications, the number of pharmacists produced is relatively smaller than in countries where the "drugstore" also sells candy, tobacco products, and many other commodities. Thus, in the United States there are more than twice as many pharmacists per capita as there are in Great Britian where the "chemist shop" dispenses solely pharmaceutical drugs.

REFERENCES

Aiken L. H. ed. *Nursing in the 1980's: Crises, Opportunities, Challenges.* Philadelphia: Lippincott, 1982.

Aiken, L. H., & Mullinix, C. F. "The Nurse Shortage." *New England Journal of Medicine, 317,* 645, 1987.

American Hospital News. "Hospitals' brace for Medicare cuts," November 12, 1990.

American Hospital News. "Hospitals' creative extender models help relieve nurse shortage," December 3, 1990.

AMA; American Medical Association. *Medical Groups in the U.S.—a Survey of Practice Characteristics 1990 Edition.* Chicago: 1990.

ANA, American Nurses Association. *Nursing Association Policy Statement.* Kansas City, MO: 1980.

ANA, American Nurses Association. *The Nursing Practice Act: Suggested State Legislation.* New York: 1981.

ANA, American Nurses Association. "Nursing Shortage Update." *Nurses, Media Backgrounder,* February 1990.

Center for Nursing. *Restructuring the Work Load: Methods and Models to Address the Nursing Shortage.* Chicago: American Hospital Association, 1989.

Colwill, J. M. "Education of the Primary Physician: A Time for Reconsideration?" *Journal of the American Medical Association, 255,* 2643, 1986.

Committee on Medical Schools & Association of American Medical Colleges in Relation to Training for Family Practice. "Planning for Comprehensive and Continuing Care of patients through Education." *Journal of Medical Education, 43,* 751, 1986.

Donabedian, A., et al. *Medical Care Chartbook,* 7th ed. Ann Arbor, MI: AUPHA Press, 1980.

Eisenberg, J. M. *Doctors' Decisions and the Cost of Medical Care.* Ann Arbor, MI: Health Administration Press, 1986.

Geyman, J. P. "Training Primary Care Physicians for the 21st Century." *Journal of the American Medical Association, 255,* 2631, 1986.

Gillis, K. D., & Wilke, R. J. "Employment Patterns of Physicians, 1983–1989." In *Socioeconomic Characteristics of Medical Practice, 1989,* ed. M. L. Gonzalez & D. W. Emmons. Chicago: American Medical Association, 1989.

Helmer, F. T. & McKnight, P. "Management strategies to minimize nursing turnover." *Health Care Management Review, 14*(1), 73, 1989.

Kalisch, P. A., & Kalisch, B. J. *The Advance of American Nursing.* Boston: Little, Brown, 1978.

Kim, M. J., McFarland G. K., and McLane, A. M., eds. *Classification of Nursing Diagnosis: Proceedings of the Fifth National Congress.* St. Louis: Mosby, 1984.

Leape, L. L., et al. "Relation Between Surgeons' Practice Volumes and Geographic Variation in the Rate of Carotid Endarterectomy." *New England Journal of Medicine, 321,* 653, 1989.

NCHS, National Center for Health Statistics. *Health: United States, 1989.* Hyattsville, MD: DHHS Pub. No. (PHS) 90-1232, 1990.

Neylan, M. "Eight Ways to Relieve the Nursing Shortage." *RNABC News,* November–December 1989, p. 5.

Premier Focus. "Nursing." Westchester, IL: Premier Hospitals Alliance, October 1990.

Record, J., et al. *Primary Care Staffing in 1990: Physician Replacement and Cost Savings.* New York: Springer Publishing, 1981.

Relman, A. S. "The Debate on Primary-Care Manpower," *New England Journal of Medicine, 299,* 1305, 1978.

Schafft, G. E., & Cawley, J. F. *The Physician Assistant.* Rockville, MD: Aspen, 1987.

Schwenk, T. L., & Wooley, F. R. "The Role of the Community-Oriented Primary Care Physician." *American Journal of Preventive Medicine, 2*(1), 49, 1986.

Secretary's Commission on Nursing. *Final Report.* Washington, DC: USDHHS, December 1988.

Stein, L. I., et al. "The Doctor-Nurse Game Revisited." *New England Journal of Medicine, 322,* 546, 1990.

Tolchin, M. "States Take up New Burdens to Pay for 'New Federalism.' " *The New York Times,* May 21, 1990, p. A1.

USNY, University of the State of New York. *Medicine Handbook.* Albany, NY: New York State Education Department, December 1989.

USNY, University of the State of New York. *Nursing Handbook.* Albany, NY: New York State Education Department, April 1990.

Wennberg, J. E. "Dealing with Medical Practice Variations: A Proposal for Action." *Health Affairs, 3,* 6, 1984.

White, K. L. "Organization and Delivery of Personal Health Services—Public Policy Issues." *Milbank Memorial Fund Quarterly,* January 1968; reprinted in *Politics and Law in Health Care Policy,* ed. J. B. McKinlay. New York: Prodist, 1973.

Chapter **5**

Government

In the United States, the government operates neither the health-care delivery system nor the health-services financing system in its entirety; government is less involved in health care than in any other industrialized country. Perhaps the most important reason for this difference is the strength of the private medical sector and its opposition to "government control and interference" (except in select areas, such as care of the sick poor, care of the mentally ill, and infectious disease control). Restricted as the government's role is compared with that in other nations, however, on an absolute scale, in terms of dollars spent, for example, it looms large. This role has developed and expanded gradually over a long period of time.

SOME HISTORY

In his preface to a seminal book of the 1940s by Bernhard J. Stern, one of the first medical sociologists, one of the noted authorities on public health of the day, W. G. Smillie, said (Stern, p. xiii):

> Our forefathers certainly had no concept of responsibility of the Federal Government, nor of the state government, for health protection of the people. This was solely a local governmental responsibility. When Benjamin Franklin wrote "Health is Wealth" in the Farmers' Almanac, he was saying that health was a commodity to be bought, to be sold, to be conserved, or to be wasted. But he considered that health conservation was the responsibility of the individual, not of government. The local community was responsible only for the protection of its citizens against the hazards of community life.
> Thus government responsibility for health protection consisted of (a) promotion of sanitation and (b) communicable disease control. The Federal Constitution, as well as the Constitutions of most of the states, contains no reference or intimation of a federal or state function in

medical care. The care of the sick poor was a local community responsibility from earliest pioneer days. This activity was assumed first by voluntary philanthropy; later, it was transferred, and became an official governmental obligation.

Professor Stern continued that line of thinking in his introduction (pp. 4–5):

> Government action in the field has traditionally been limited to the care of the indigent and has been dominated in its scope and administration by the restraining influences of the parochial poor laws. Gradually, and especially after the passage of the Social Security Act and during [World War II], government medical care has increasingly been furnished to some nonindigent groups. New patterns of government medical care are being formulated and the role of local, state, and federal governments in the field is changing. . . . The attitudes of the medical profession and of the public toward government medical programs will determine whether these resources are to be used progressively to distribute whether these resources are to be used progressively to distribute more medical care of higher quality of the American people.

Government at all levels in the United States is much more heavily involved in the health-care system in both degree and kind in 1991 than it was in 1946. Consider, for example, such initiatives as Medicare and Medicaid, new regulatory powers, and support of biomedical research and health professions education. But certain characteristics have remained unchanged. They are most significant. To quote Smillie again (Stern, p. xiv): "Practically all governmental procedures in medical care stem from the original local community responsibility for the care of the sick poor, and many of our great municipal hospitals, clinics, and health services of today still bear the stigma of pauperism."

The pauper stigma, that "poor equals bad" and that poverty is the fault of the poor, is still attached to much government activity in direct-care delivery (although certain health department services have managed to escape the taint). It is rooted in the Protestant ethic, which held people directly accountable for their lives. The legal implementation of the Protestant ethic goes back at least as far as the Elizabethan Poor Laws in England (de Schweinitz).

While in our society today some may accept socioeconomic explanations of why some people are well off and others destitute, the attitudes of many toward the proper role of government in health care are still colored by old values and prejudices (Jonas, 1986). In rallying broad public support for its consistent policy of cutting programs aimed at helping the poor (Hayward; Igelhart, 1985a, 1985b), the Reagan administration was apparently able to tap many of these values and prejudices. These cuts appeared to have a negative impact on health services for, and the health of, the poor and minorities (Bindman; NCHS; Wenneker et al.).

Many questions remain about the role of government in health, some of which have resonated for decades. In his preface to the landmark report of the Institute of Medicine's Committee on The Future of Public Health, Dr. Richard Remington summarized them well (IOM, pp. v–vi):

> But what is the most appropriate nature of that governmental presence? How should government's role relate to that of the private sector? How should governmental responsibility for public health be apportioned among local, state, and federal levels? Should government be the health care provider of last resort or does it have a greater responsibility? Should public health consist only of a necessary residuum of activities not met by private providers? How should governmental activities directed toward the maintenance of an environment conducive to health be apportioned among various agencies? But above all, just what is public health? What does it include and what does it exclude? Based on an appropriate definition, what kinds of programs and agencies should be constructed to meet the needs and demands of the public, which is often resistant to an increasing role, or at least an increasing cost, of government?

THE CONSTITUTIONAL BASIS OF GOVERNMENT AUTHORITY IN HEALTH CARE

To understand government operations in the health-care system, it is essential to understand the structure of the government itself.* A basic principle of the Constitution is that sovereign power is to be shared between federal and state governments, a principle called federalism. At its heart, the Constitution is an agreement between the original 13 states to delegate some of their inherent powers to the federal government. As part of this agreement, in the Tenth Amendment to the Constitution, the states (and through them the people at large) explicitly reserved to themselves the rest: "The powers not

---

*The *Public Health Law Manual*, by Frank P. Grad (1990), and *Health and the Law*, by Tom Christoffel (1982), are valuable guides to the legal basis of government activity in health care and to the many legal procedures involved in the enforcement of public health law.

delegated to the United States by the Constitution, nor prohibited by it to the states, are reserved to the states respectively, or to the people."

Since it is not explicitly mentioned in the Constitution, among the powers reserved to the states is the *police power*, which forms the basis of the states' role in health (Mustard, pp. 17–21). As Grad points out (p. 10):

> In the states, government authority to regulate for the protection of public health and to provide health services is based on the "police power"—that is, the power to provide for the health, safety, and welfare of the people. It is not necessary that his power be expressly stated, because it is a plenary power that every sovereign government has, simply by virtue of being a sovereign government. For purposes of the police power, the state governments—which antedate the federal government—are sovereign governments. . . . The exercise of the police power is really what government is about. It defines government.

Among the states' other inherent powers is delegation of their authority. The states have used it to create a third tier of government, local government. Most states have delegated some of their health powers to that tier. The constitutional basis of the federal government's health authority is found in the powers to tax and spend to provide for the general welfare, and to regulate interstate and foreign commerce (see Article I, Section 8 of the Constitution; Grad, pp. 11–15).

The other basic constitutional principle affecting health and health services is the "separation of powers." The Constitution divides the sovereign powers of the federal government among three branches of government: executive, legislative, and judicial. Under separation of powers, each branch of the federal government has its own authority and responsibility, spelled out in the Constitution. Further, the Constitution spells out curbs on the powers of each branch exercised by the other two, the system of "checks and balances." (One very important check on the power of both the federal legislative and executive branches, judicial review of the constitutionality of their actions, is not found in the Constitution, however. It was established early in the nineteeth century by the third chief justice of the Supreme Court, John Marshall. It has become an accepted part of U.S. constitutional law and procedure only because the other two branches have granted the Court that authority in practice and have followed its determinations.)

The state governments follow fairly closely the tripartite form of government, with checks and balances. At the local level, the boundaries between branches become blurred at times. For example, in some suburban and rural areas, the local chief executive officer presides over the local legislative body. Nevertheless, in most jurisdictions, separation of powers is a major principle of government.

THE FUNCTIONS OF GOVERNMENT IN THE U.S. HEALTH CARE SYSTEM

The Legislative Branch

At each level of government—federal, state, and local—each of the three branches of government has responsibility and authority for health and health services. Legislatures create the laws that establish the means to safeguard the public's health in matters ranging from the assurance of a pure water supply to protecting the health of workers in their places of employment. They enact the legal framework within which the health-care functions, deciding which individuals and institutions are authorized to deliver what services to which persons under what conditions and requirements.

Legislatures may impose certain requirements for planning and development of the system (see Chapter 6). If the government is to participate in health-care financing (see Chapters 7 and 8), directly deliver services (see Chapters 2 and 3) or support research efforts, the legislature must first establish those programs.

The Judiciary

The judicial branches at the three levels of government have important powers relating to health and health services. However, they cannot apprehend transgressors, prosecute them, or carry out punishment on their own. Thus, they must work in concert with the law-enforcement arms of the executive branches under the authority granted to them by their legislatures. Together, the judicial and executive branches form the civil and criminal justice systems.

The judiciary supports the work of the other branches of government. For example, although it is the state legislature that creates a licensing law for physicians and the executive branch that administers it, it is the judicial system that determines the guilt or innocence of a person charged with practicing medicine without a license. The judicial system adjudicates disputes arising from the provision of health services (e.g., malpractice litigation). It protects the rights of individuals under the due-process and equal-protection clauses of the Fifth and Fourteenth Amendments to the Constitution. The criminal justice system as a whole plays a vital role in the safeguarding of the public's health. For example, it enforces sanitary-protection and pollution-control legislation.

The Executive Branch

The term *government in health care* usually refers to the executive branch, which delivers health-care services, drafts and enforces provider regulations, and administers financing programs. In the remainder of this chapter, the term *government* refers to the executive branch.

Provision of Personal Health Services

At the federal level, personal health services are provided for the most part to categories of persons: members of the uniformed services and their families, Native Americans, and veterans, for example. State governments provide personal health services for the most part to persons who have specific diseases, primarily mental illness and tuberculosis. Local government personal health services are generally for the lower socioeconomic class and the medically indigent.

There are occasional overlaps. For example, it is the federal government that provides care for those afflicted with Hansen's disease (leprosy), and it operates St. Elizabeth's Hospital, a mental institution in the District of Columbia. Governments at all levels provide health services for occupants of their prisons.

Provision of Community Health Services

Government at all levels is the major provider of the traditional "public health" services such as pure water supply and sanitary sewage disposal, food and drug inspection and regulation, communicable disease control (e.g., immunization and the control of sexually transmitted diseases), and vital statistics and public health laboratory work. Certain community health activities are shared with the private sector. For example, in public health education, voluntary agencies such as the American Cancer Society and the American Heart Association are important participants. Private refuse collectors do much of the solid-waste collection. Private organizations like the Sierra Club and the Natural Resources Defense Council are active in environmental protection. Private institutions play a vital role in health-sciences education and research.

Health Services Financing

Government participates in the financing system in three ways (see also Chapter 7). First, it pays for its own programs, both personal and community. This can be direct, as in operating the federal government's veterans' hospitals or a municipal hospital serving primarily the poor, or indirect, as in the federal government's grants to state governments to help support care in state mental hospitals. Likewise, state and federal governments spend directly to collect vital statistics, and they give money to local governments to help them in so doing.

Second, by grants and contracts to nongovernmental agencies (and in certain cases, other governmental agencies), governments support other types of health-related programs; for example, in biomedical research and medical education. Third, governments pay providers on an item-of-service basis for the delivery of care to third parties under such programs as Medicare and Medicaid (see Chapter 7). Federal, state, and local public funds accounted for about 42 percent of national health expenditures in 1988 (see Chapter 7).

THE FEDERAL GOVERNMENT AND THE PROVISION OF HEALTH SERVICES

Many federal agencies are involved in the delivery of personal and community health services. The U.S. Department of Health and Human Services (USDHHS) is the most important federal actor in health. The are two other Federal agencies with major health-services responsibilities: the Departments of Veterans Affairs and Defense. Other federal agencies with significant health-related responsibilities include the Department of Agriculture (nutrition policy, meat and poultry inspection, food stamps), the Environmental Protection Agency, and the Department of Labor (the Occupational Safety and Health Act).

USDHHS

The Department of Health and Human Services has five major operating divisions (USDHHS, 1990a): the Public Health Service, the

Health Care Financing Administration, the Social Security Administration, the Office of Human Development Services, and the Family Support Administration. The first two are the principal health agencies, although each of the other three has certain health responsibilities.

Public Health Service

The assistant secretary for health directs the Public Health Service (PHS). The Public Health Service has a long and proud history, dating to a 1798 act creating the Marine Hospital Service (MHS) (Mustard, pp 23–81; Schmeckebier, chap. 1; Stern, pp. 145–154). In 1878, Congress added foreign quarantine responsibilities to the work of the MHS. This lead in 1889 to the development of a quasi-military personnel system, the "commissioned corps" of the PHS. The corps was made up largely of career medical people. Its commander is the surgeon general of the United States.

The PHS continued to gain responsibilities over the years. Following the end of World War II, the PHS grew rapidly, with the passage of the Hospital Survey and Construction Act of 1946 (Hill-Burton Act); the vigorous growth of the National Institutes of Health; the creation of the Communicable Disease Center in Atlanta (later, the Centers for Disease Control); and the development of drug-abuse control, mental retardation, mental health centers, and comprehensive health-planning activities.

As of 1990, the PHS had eight major divisions (USDHHS, 1990a): the Health Resources and Services Administration; the Centers for Disease Control; the Food and Drug Administration; the National Institutes of Health; the Alcohol, Drug Abuse, and Mental Health Administration; the Indian Health Service; the Agency for Toxic Substances and Disease Registry; and the Agency for Health Care Policy and Research. The PHS thus has a wide variety of functions: regulator, provider of direct personal and community health services, provider of financial support for a variety of health services through the grant and contract mechanism, research agency, the principal federal supporter of biomedical research in nongovernment agencies.

The Health Resources and Services Administration (HRSA) runs the direct-service programs of DHHS; supports efforts to improve the education and use of the nation's health personnel; supports efforts to improve health-care programs, especially for underserved populations; attempts to improve the use of health facilities; aids in increasing the number of minorities in the health professions; administers the National Health Service Corps (which provides financial aid to selected medical students in return for a service commitment from them for work in underserved communities upon the completion of their training); and participates in the AIDS-control program in a variety of ways.

The Centers for Disease Control (CDC) is the national public health agency primarily responsible for prevention efforts. Its programs are aimed at preventing and controlling disease, directing foreign and interstate quarantine operations, developing programs for health education and health promotion, improving the performance of clinical laboratories, and developing the standards necessary to insure safe and healthful working conditions for all working people. Through the National Center for Health Statistics it collects and publishes a wide variety of vital, health, and health-services data. It maintains the nation's reference laboratories and supports laboratory training programs. It also awards project grants to state and local health agencies to support immunization, particularly for children.

The task of the Food and Drug Administration (FDA) is to protect the public against food, drug, and medical-devices hazards, and to assure drug potency and effectiveness. Thus, the FDA regulates prescription drugs and over-the-counter medications, biological products, and human blood and its derivatives. The focus is on the assurance of the efficacy and safety of a product before marketing, and on the assurance of continuing quality after approval. Medical devices are regulated in a similar manner. Radiological equipment is also regulated to control radiation exposure to the public. In addition, the FDA has responsibilities in veterinary medicine and toxicology.

The regulatory programs of the FDA, especially those focusing on the efficacy and safety of drugs and medical devices, are sometimes controversial. Industry leaders state that the entry of useful drugs to the market is at times unnecessarily delayed by a lengthy and expensive approval process. By and large, however, this regulatory program has strong support from the public and Congress. They recall, for example, the Thalidomide disaster. It seems unlikely that it will be substantially weakened. (See Addendun I to this chapter for a discussion of the pharmaceutical industry.)

Through its multiple institutes such as the National Cancer Institute and the National Heart, Lung, and Blood Institute, the National Institutes of Health (NIH) is responsible for supporting and carrying out biomedical research. Its primary mission focuses on basic biomedical research at the organ-system, tissue, cellular, and subcellular level. Although other federal agencies also support biomedical research, the NIH alone accounts for about two-thirds of the federal investment in it. NIH has its own (intramural) research program on its campus in Bethesda, Maryland, and provides funds for research at many other institutions around the country through (extramural) grants and contracts. NIH also fosters research by supporting training, resource development, and construction.

The Alcohol, Drug Abuse, and Mental Health Administration (ADAMHA) is divided into three parts: the National Institute on Alcohol Abuse and Alcoholism, the National Institute on Drug Abuse, and the National Institute of Mental Health. The agency conducts clinical and biomedical research in its laboratories; funds extramural research, research training, and prevention programs through grants and contracts; and provides technical assistance and information about the health problems that it addresses.

The Indian Health Service provides health care for about 1 million Native Americans in the continental 48 states and Alaska who live on or near traditional tribal lands. Health services include hospital, ambulatory, preventive, rehabilitative care, and community sanitation. The Indian Health Service has a system of about 50 hospitals, 80 health centers, 750 smaller health stations, satellite clinics, and a network of providers working on contract.

The Agency for Toxic Substances and Disease Registry is a recent creation in the PHS. It "seeks to mitigate the adverse health effects that may accompany exposure to hazardous substances in the environment" (USDHHS, 1990a). The newest PHS component is the Agency for Health Care Policy and Research. It "conducts and supports studies aimed at improving the quality and cost-effectiveness of the nation's health care delivery system" (USDHHS, 1990a).

Office of Disease Prevention and Health Promotion

An important health agency found in the Office of the Assistant Secretary for Health but not a formal part of the PHS is the Office of Disease Prevention and Health Promotion (ODPHP) (McGinniss). A deputy assistant secretary of health heads ODPHP. Its primary responsibility is to strengthen the health-promotion and disease-prevention activities of DHHS in collaboration with the PHS and other DHHS agencies.

In 1989, ODPHP published *The Guide to Clinical Preventive Services* (USPSTF), the product of the work of the U.S. Preventive Services Task Force. Over a three-year period, that body reviewed and evaluated about 170 clinical preventive interventions in common use. In 1990, ODPHP published *Healthy People 2000: National Health Promotion and Disease Prevention Objectives* (USDHHS, 1990b) for the year 2000, a set of goals and specific health objectives in 22 priority areas ranging from exercise to cancer prevention, from environmental health to immunization, for the health-care system and our people as a whole to strive for.

Among its other undertakings, the ODPHP operates the National Health Information Center, has cooperative agreements with a variety of private agencies to implement the Healthy People 2000 initiative, and works with a number of private entities to further various health-promotion–disease-prevention activities ranging from worksite wellness programs to the improvement of nutrition.

The Department of Veterans Affairs

The Department of Veterans Affairs (DVA) was formed from the old Veterans Administration in 1989 (Derwinski). After military service, the U.S. veteran becomes entitled to a remarkably broad range of health services. If a disorder is connected with military service, its care is a responsibility of the DVA for life. For any other disorder, health care is available as so long as the veteran states it would cause him financial "hardship" to obtain the care privately. Among the nations of the world, the United States is unique in supporting so broad a range of health services for veterans, a fact doubtless related to the lack of national health insurance for the general population.

The DVA operates the largest centrally directed hospital and clinic system in the United States. In 1989 about 27.1 million veterans, 11 percent of the population, were eligible to receive at least a portion of their health care from the DVA (DVA, p. 17). The origins of the DVA medical services can be traced to a 1776 report of a committee of the Continental Congress. It was established "to consider what provision ought to be made for such as are wounded or disabled in the land or sea service, and report a plan for that purpose" (*Journals of the Contintental Congress*, p. 469). The committee recommended the establishment of a pension system for disabled veterans. (Precedent for such a system can be traced back to an act of the English Parliament in its 1592–1593 session. That act provided relief for veterans of the

1588 war with Spain. On this continent, as early as 1636 the Plymouth Colony undertook to care for soldiers disabled in the Pequot War.) The federal government took on the responsibility in 1789.

Following the Civil War, the federal government established the National Military and Naval Home. It was to care for Union Army veterans with service-connected disabilities causing "economic distress." Later, the facilities were made available to all veterans, and the qualifying "economic distress" did not necessarily have to be related to military service.

After World War I, the Public Health Service hospitals for merchant seamen were assigned the responsibility of caring for the large influx of disabled veterans. The system was expanded greatly by the addition of certain military hospitals and the construction of new ones. By June 1920, there were 11,639 beds in 52 hospitals. In 1922, the veterans' hospitals were transferred to the Veterans Bureau, which became the Veterans Administration in 1930.

In fiscal year 1988, the DVA was operating 172 medical centers with about 74,000 hospital beds. This number was down sharply from the 90,154 beds in service in 1978. There were 60 satellite or independent clinics, 233 outpatient clinics, 119 nursing-home units, 28 domiciliaries, and 194 Readjustment Counselling Vet Centers (Derwinski, pp. 7–8). There were about 202,000 full-time equivalents on staff. There was at least one DVA hosptial in every state except Alaska and Hawaii where veterans are hospitalized in civilian facilities under contract. There is no VA hospital in Puerto Rico; veterans are handled as in Alaska and Hawaii. In 1988, the DVA's annual health-care budget was over $10.5 billion, the bulk of it going to medical care. There were over 1.2 million inpatients and 23.2 million outpatient visits to DVA facilities.

A *veteran* is defined as anyone who served 90 days or more in an armed service, but a veteran must have received an honorable or general discharge to be automatically eligible. Thus, there is a "moral means test" based on discharge status. Among those holding honorable or general discharges, there are four overlapping groups of veterans eligible to receive DVA medical care: (1) veterans with service-connected disabilities or certain other qualifying characteristics such as having been exposed to herbicides in Vietnam; (2) recipients of DVA pensions; (3) veterans 65 and older; (4) veterans meeting certain income means tests (DVA, pp. 38–47). Veterans other than those in categories 1 and 2 may have to pay a portion of the charges for their care. The DVA estimates that about 55 percent of veterans are eligible to receive health benefits (Derwinski, p. 11).

In the late 1980s, the major challenge facing the health-care system of the DVA is the rapid aging of the veteran population. In 1988, 24 percent of veterans were over 65, 44 percent 45 to 64, and 33 percent under 45. The corresponding figures from the general population 20 and older were 17 percent, 26 percent, and 56 percent.

Department of Defense (DOD)

The army, navy, air force, and marines each has its own network of hospitals, clinics, and field posts. All DOD health personnel are members of the military, salaried according to their military ranks (without relation to the services they render). The same basic structure prevails in war or peace. Health promotion and disease prevention are emphasized and integrated with the delivery of treatment.

According to the comptroller general (1979, p. 1), military medicine's four principal objectives are

1. To maintain physically and mentally fit service personnel and trained health personnel to support combat, contingency, and mobilization plans.
2. To provide care and treatment capabilities in a theater of operations and in the United States for combat casualties.
3. To provide health services for dependents of soldiers, retired career service personnel and their dependents, and dependents and survivors of deceased career service personnel.
4. To provide a major incentive for soldiers, including health professionals, to select military service as a career.

Thus, through its own facilities or through contracting arrangements, DOD provides health services to members of the armed forces, their dependents, surviving dependents of servicepeople killed while on active duty, and military retirees and *their* dependents. (Service personnel are eligible for retirement benefits after a minimum of 20 years of service. The health-services part of that package is in addition to those of the DVA for which they may be eligible.) In 1990, about 9.25 million people in the United States, or about 4 percent of the population, received all or most of their health care under the auspices of the DOD (ASD).

Care for persons other than uniformed servicepeople is sometimes provided at military facilities. In addition, the Civilian Health and Medical Program of the Uniformed Services (CHAMPUS) is an important medical-care resource for civilian beneficiaries (ASD).

CHAMPUS is a reimbursement system that pays for the costs of care in the private sector. Theoretically, all persons potentially eligible under CHAMPUS must first seek care from a military medical facility and be unable to obtain it for one reason or another.

An unusual aspect of military medical departments is that they are charged not only with providing a full range of direct health services but also with providing for the environmental health of their communities. This combination of administrative responsibilities for personal and community preventive and treatment services is rarely found elsewhere in the U.S. health-care system.

Other Federal Departments

Many federal departments have some health responsibilities. For example, the U.S. Department of Agriculture (USDA) provides some health services for agricultural families and farm workers, control programs for animal diseases, and plant health services. The USDA also operates nutrition services, such as the Women and Infants Care (WIC) program, school breakfast and lunch programs, and the food-stamp program. It conducts research on the nutrient composition of foods, food consumption, and nutritional requirements. In cooperation with the USDHHS, it periodically issues dietary guidelines. It supervises food-safety regulations in cooperation with the FDA and grades meats and other foods for consumers. It also has programs in nutrition education and research.

Focusing on preventive activities in the workplace, the Occupational Safety and Health Administration (OSHA) is part of the Department of Labor. OSHA uses criteria developed by the National Institute of Occupational Safety and Health (NIOSH), part of the CDC, to set national standards for occupational safety and health (Brock and Tyson). The major responsibilities of OSHA are to develop workplace health and safety standards, to enforce and gain compliance with the standards, to engage in education and training, to help the states in occupational safety and health matters, and to aid business in meeting OSHA requirements. There are a few industries that are not covered by OSHA; for example, the health and safety of miners is the province of the Bureau of Mines in the Department of the Interior.

The Environmental Protection Agency (EPA) is an independent (nondepartmental) agency that has major responsibilities for the control of air and water quality and pollution, solid-waste disposal, pesticide contamination, radiation hazards, electromagnetic pollution, and toxic substances (EPA, 1988, 1989). The EPA conducts research on air, water, and land pollution-control technology and the effects of pollution on humans, develops criteria and issues national standards for pollutants, and enforces compliance with these standards.

THE STATE GOVERNMENTS' ROLE IN HEALTH SERVICES

As at the federal level, at the state level many different agencies are involved in health services.* In fact, in most states departments other than the state health department provide two of the important health-related functions: mental illness services (by the department of mental health) and Medicaid (by the welfare department). The licensing authority for health personnel sometimes resides in the education department; vocational rehabilitation in a special agency; occupational health in the labor department; environmental protection in a separate department; and school health with local boards of education. Most states also have a board of health, usually appointed by the governor, which has varying administrative, policy, and advisory functions.

In the 1920s, political struggles with private practitioners, (referred to in Chapter 3) led to a limitation of service responsibilities for state and local health departments. Haven Emerson, a leading public health official of the time, defined the "Basic Six" services appropriate for departments of public health: vital statistics, public health laboratories, communicable disease control, environmental sanitation, maternal and child health, and public health education (Wilson & Neuhauser, p. 204). Since World War II, governments have vastly expanded the responsibilities of both state and local departments of health to include regulation and quality control, rate setting, institutional licensure, and planning. And as noted above, state and local health-related activities outside of the health departments have expanded.

State Health Services

Not all states call their principal health agency the health department. Thus, the Association of State and Territorial Health Officials (ASTHO) established the designation State Health Agency (SHA),

---

*A comprehensive review of state and local (as well as federal) public health activities, with an extensive bibliography, is in appendix A of *The Future of Public Health* (IOM). See also *Public Health Agencies 1990* (PHF).

defined as "the agency vested with primary responsibility for public health within their jurisdictions" (ASTHO, 1983, p. vii). ASTHO defined a health program as "a set of identifiable services organized to solve health related problems or to meet specific health or health related needs, provided to or on behalf of the public, by or under the direction of an organizational entity in a State Health Agency, and for which reasonably accurate estimates of expenditures can be made" (ASTHO, 1980, p. vii). Using this definition, ASTHO identified six program areas for SHAs: "personal health, environmental health, health resources, laboratory, general administration and services, and funds to local health departments not allocated to program areas" (ASTHO, 1980, p. 9). While the number is still six, the content is much expanded beyond that of the "Basic Six."

A significant number of SHAs report having identifiable public health services in the following areas (some services are provided by local health departments) (ASTHO 1980, 1983; PHF):

- Maternal and child health, including prenatal and postnatal services, family planning, immunization, and well-baby care.
- Public and personal health education.
- Communicable disease control, including immunization, tuberculosis and venereal disease control, epidemiology, and laboratory services.
- Dental health, emphasizing preventive services.
- Handicapped children's services.
- Environmental health, including consumer protection, sanitation, air and water quality control, waste management, occupational health and safety, and radiation control.
- Health planning and resources development, regulations and statistics.
- Laboratory, including analytical services and laboratory improvement.

Personal Health Services

Most SHAs have programs in maternal and child health, communicable disease control, chronic disease control, and dental health. Many operate programs for handicapped children, home care, and speech, occupational, or physical therapy. Although state public health services are available in theory to the general population, according to an ASTHO survey (1980, p. 65; see also PHF, p. 1) most programs were targeted to persons with low incomes. In about 80 percent of

SHAs, local health departments participate in the delivery of at least some of their services.

Environmental Health Programs

At the federal level, many agencies are active in environmental health. At the state level, the picture is even more complicated. Under federal environmental health law, the governor of each state has designated a "lead environmental agency." In most it is *not* the SHA; it is usually an environmental-protection or natural-resources agency. Nevertheless, in some of the states in which the SHA is not the designated lead environmental agency, it still has important environmental health functions (e.g., in sanitation, pure water supply, and sanitary sewage disposal).

The major environmental health programs carried out by SHAs (and non-SHA environmental protection agencies) are:

- Consumer protection and sanitation: food and milk control, substance control and product safety, sanitation of health care facilities and other institutions, housing and recreational sanitation, and vector and zoonotic disease control.
- Water-quality services: public and individual water supply and individual sewage disposal, with public water pollution-control services usually provided by an agency other than the SHA.
- Radiation control.
- Occupational health and safety, accident prevention, and noise-pollution control.
- Solid and hazardous waste management.
- Environmental health training.
- Environmental health-planning, design, and impact studies.

Health Resources

Among the oldest of public health functions is the collection and analysis of vital and health statistics. In recent years, SHAs have expanded (in some states greatly expanded) their activities in such areas as health planning, health-resources development, and health-resources regulation (see also Chapter 6).

Licensing

Licensing, particularly of physicians, is a basic governmental function in health care. It is a good example of the involvement of all three branches of government in health: the legislatures enact the statutes; the executive branches administer them; and the courts interpret and enforce them. Licensing of individuals determines who may deliver what kinds of health services and establishes minimum standards for licensure qualification. Licensing of institutions also sets minimum standards for the facility and its personnel. The licensing authority is one of the most significant of the health powers of the states. The way it is used is a major determinant of the character of the United States' health-care delivery system.

The medical licensing system gives physicians tight control over the central product of the health-care system: medical services (see Chapter 7). By exercising this control, physicians largely determine the structure of the health-care system: how it is organized, the types and functions of the institutions, and the powers of the several categories of personnel who work in it.

THE LOCAL GOVERNMENTS' ROLE IN HEALTH SERVICES

It is difficult to speak authoritatively about local health departments. First, there is no generally accepted definition of a local health department (LHD). Second, there is no national roster or ongoing annual reporting system for local health departments. However, a series of studies of them undertaken by Miller and his colleagues in the 1970s provided much useful information (Miller, et al., 1979; Miller & Moos).

Following a survey of what state health officers considered local health departments, Miller and his colleagues developed a definition of an LHD (Miller et al., 1977, p. 931): "An administrative and service unit of local or state government, concerned with health, employing at least one full time person and carrying some responsibility for the health of a jurisdiction smaller than a state."

The National Public Health Program Reporting System (NPHPRS) of ASTHO came up with a different definition of an LHD (ASTHO, 1980, p. 36) in 1990, also subscribed to by the Public Health Foundation (PHF, p. 143):

> An official (governmental) public health agency which is in whole or in part responsible to a sub-state governmental entity. In addition, a local health department must meet these criteria: (A) It has a staff of one or more full time professional public health employees (e.g., public health nurse, sanitarian); (B) it delivers public health services; (C) it serves a

definable geographic area; and (D) it has identifiable expenditures and/ or budget in the political subdivision(s) which it serves.

Most LHDs are based on single local jurisdictions: city, county, town, village, and so forth. Many LHDs are limited to the Basic Six, although in recent years some have become involved in the direct delivery of ambulatory services to the poor. Following the state and federal models, local health services are also provided by various agencies other than health departments. For example, cities and counties are likely to place their hospitals for the poor (see Chapter 3) and their mental health services in separate agencies. Water supply, sanitary sewage and solid-waste disposal, and pollution control are also likely to be in separate agencies if the private sector does not handle them.

Commonly, LHDs provide one or more of the following services: immunization, environmental surveillance, tuberculosis control, maternal and child health, school health, venereal disease control, chronic-disease control, home care, family planning, ambulatory care, and health-code enforcement. Thus, the LHDs, in cooperation with SHAs and other state agencies, particularly in environmental health, are the backbone of the system for providing public health and preventive services.

LHDs and Ambulatory Care

Despite advances in public perceptions of what is right and declining opposition from the private medical sector, the provision of general ambulatory-care services by LHDs remains a controversial matter. The controversy is over the ability of local health departments to mount such services. Some have expressed optimism that this change in role can be accomplished (Miller; Roemer). Miller sees local health departments as having major responsibility for the delivery of direct social and medical services to the poor.

Others feel that given the history of local health departments (with their bureaucratic administrative structure and their close involvement with politically sensitive, financially pressed local governments, along with continuing opposition from the private sector in some communities, except in certain unique circumstances), the chances are limited that much headway will be made in this direction (Jonas, 1977, chaps. 5, 7). The goal should be the creation of a comprehensive national health program (see Chapter 8), so that there are no gaps in medical services that local health departments must stretch to fill. Then they can better deal with the health-promotion–disease-prevention tasks for which they have primary responsibility.

In 1983, then commissioner of the New York City Health Department David Sencer, put the prevention-oriented view of the local health department's role this way (p. 89):

> Given today's needs, the ideal urban health department should: (1) treat the community, not the individual, as the patient; (2) have the primary responsibility in its community for assuring primary prevention with the capability of providing such services if others are not so doing; (3) divorce itself from all curative programs except those that are themselves a means of primary prevention; . . . and (5) possess the technical expertise that is a prerequisite for leadership.

Dr. Sencer also stated, "The local health department should provide those services that others have not, will not, should not, or cannot provide" (p. 91). A "have-not" service is immunization; a "will-not" service (in many cases) is occupational health; a "should-not" service (because of lack of technical expertise) is a public health laboratory; and a "cannot" service is surveillance, which Dr. Sencer describes as "the backbone of the health department" (p. 92).

To this list one might add that in the current era local health departments should take the lead in promoting health promotion and disease prevention on a communitywide basis. For example, they should be advocating the creation of smoke-free workplaces, the banning of cigarette vending machines as proposed by the secretary of Health and Human Services, healthier eating habits, and regular exercise.

Only where the local government does not have a hospitals department or its equivalent and other arrangements cannot be made should health departments even consider providing direct treatment service for the poor. To do so sops up scarce money for community health services. Further, those who agree with Dr. Sencer say, it draws the attention of public health officers from those controversies that arise from their handling of increasingly complicated community preventive-services issues.

PROBLEMS IN PUBLIC HEALTH

State and local public health services, and indeed federal ones too, face many problems. Perhaps the current state of affairs was best summarized by the Committee on the Future of Public Health (IOM, pp. 1–2):

Many of the major improvements in the health of the American people have been accomplished through public health measures. . . . But the public has come to take the success of public health for granted. . . . This nation has lost sight of its public health goals and has allowed the system of public health activities to fall into disarray.

Public health is what we, as a society, do collectively to assure the conditions in which people can be healthy. . . . Many problems demonstrate the need to protect the nation's health through effective, organized, and sustained effort by the public sector. . . . The current state of our abilities for effective public health action . . . is cause for national concern. . . . We have slackened our public health vigilance nationally, and the health of the public is unnecessarily threatened as a result. . . .

Successes as great as those of the past are still possible, but not without public concern and concerted action to restore America's public health capacity. This volume envisions the future of public health, analyzes the current situation and how it developed, and presents a plan of action that will, in the committee's judgement, provide a solid foundation for a strong public health capability throughout the nation.

The committee's report is commended to those readers who are concerned with the future of public health in the United States.

CONCLUSION

While government is heavily involved in the health-care system in the United States, U.S. politics and the U.S. economic system significantly limit that involvement. Government provides the legal underpinning for the system through the licensing laws. It regulates the financial workings of the system and its quality of care. Government is also a direct financier and a direct provider of service. It is preeminent in community health services and plays an important part in supporting health-sciences education and research.

However, the resistance to "government interference in the practice of medicine" is still prominent among private medical practitioners. In many laws governing the health-care system (for example, the Social Security amendments establishing the Medicare program), such interference is expressly prohibited. Most providers (often gudgingly) recognize the reality that government is already heavily involved in the practice of medicine. They welcome participation in certain critical areas: licensing; care of the mentally ill, the tubercular, and the poor; and community health services. But it is likely that the questions about the proper role of government in health summarized so well by Dr. Remington at the beginning of this chapter (p. 87) cannot be fruitfully resolved until the place and the power of the private medical sector in the health-care system as a whole is redefined.

REFERENCES

ASD, Assistant Secretary of Defense for Health Affairs. *Report on the Reorganization of Military Health Care.* Washington, DC, June 1990.

ASTHO, Association of State and Territorial Health Officials. *Comprehensive National Public Health Programs, of State and Territorial Health Agencies, Fiscal Year 1978.* Silver Springs, MD, 1980.

ASTHO. *Public Health Programs, 1981.* Kensington, MD, 1983.

Bindman, A. B., et al. "A Public Hospital Closes." *Journal of the American Medical Association, 264,* 2899, 1990.

Brock, W. E., & Tyson, P. R. *All About OSHA.* Washington, DC: Government Printing Office, 1985.

Christoffel, T. *Health and the Law.* New York: Free Press, 1982.

Comptroller General. *Military Medicine Is in Trouble.* Washington, DC: Government Printing Office, 1979.

Derwinski, E. J. *Annual Report, 1988.* Washington, DC: Department of Veterans Affairs, July 1989.

de Schweinitz, K. *England's Road to Social Security.* New York, 1943; reprinted, A. S. Barnes, 1961.

DVA, Department of Veterans' Affairs. *Federal Benefits for Veterans and Dependents.* Washington, DC, January 1990.

EPA, Environmental Protection Administration. *Environmental Progress and Challenges: EPA's Update.* Washington, DC: Government Printing Office, 1988.

EPA. *Your Guide to the United States Environmental Protection Agency.* Washington, DC: EPA Office of Public Affairs, 1989.

Grad, F. *The Public Health Law Manual,* 2nd ed. Washington, DC: American Public Health Association, 1990.

Hayward, R. R., et al. "Inequities in Health Services Among Insured Americans." *New England Journal of Medicine, 318,* 1507, 1988.

Health Resources and Services Administration. *A Profile,* Rockville, MD, April 1990.

Igelhart, J. K. "The Administration's Assault on Domestic Spending and the Threat to Health Care programs." *New England Journal of Medicine, 312,* 525, 1985a.

Igelhart, J. K. "Medical Care for the Poor—a Growing Problem." *New England Journal of Medicine, 313,* 59, 1985b.

IOM, Institute of Medicine. *The Future of Public Health.* Washington, DC, 1988.

Jonas, S. *Quality Control of Ambulatory Care: A Task for Health Departments.* New York: Springer Publishing Co., 1977.

Jonas, S. "On Homelessness and the American Way." *American Journal of Public Health, 76,* 1084, 1986.

Journals of the Continental Congress, Vol. 5.

McGinniss, J. M. *ODPHP Director's Report.* Washington, DC, January 1990.

Miller, C. A., "An Agenda for Public Health Departments," *Journal of Public Health Policy, 6,* 158, 1985.

Miller, C. A., et al. "A Survey of Local Public Health Departments and Their Directors." *American Journal of Public Health, 67,* 931, 1977.

Miller, C. A., et al. "A Study of Local Health Departments." *Bulletin of the Association of Public Health Physicians, 26,* 1, 1979.

Miller, C. A., & Moos, M. K. *Local Health Departments: Fifteen Case Studies.* Washington, DC: American Public Health Association, 1981.

Mustard, H. S. *Government in Public Health.* New York: Commonwealth Fund, 1945.

NCHS, National Center for Health Statistics. "Advance Report of Final Mortality Statistics." *Monthly Vital Statistics Report, 39*(7), suppl., November 28, 1990.

PHF, Public Health Foundation. *Public Health Agencies 1990: An Inventory of Programs and Block Grant Expenditures.* Washington, DC: Public Health Foundation, June 1990.

Roemer, M. I. "From Poor Beginnings, the Growth of Primary Care." *Hospitals,* March 1, 1975, p. 38.

Schmeckebier, L. F. *The Public Health Service.* Balitmore, MD: Johns Hopkins University Press, 1923.

Sencer, D. J. "Major Urban Health Departments: The Ideal and the Real." *Health Affairs, 2*(4), 88, 1983.

Stern, B. J. *Medical Services by Government: Local, State and Federal.* New York: Commonwealth Fund, 1946.

USDHHS, U.S. Department of Health and Human Services. *This is HHS.* Washington, DC, 1990a.

USDHHS. *Health People 2000: National Health Promotion and Disease Prevention Objectives.* Washington DC: 1990b.

USPSTF, United States Preventive Services Task Force. *The Guide to Clinical Preventive Services.* Baltimore, MD: Williams and Wilkins, 1989.

Wenneker, M. B., et al. "The Association of Payer With Utilization of Cardiac Procedures in Massachusetts." *Journal of the American Medical Association, 264,* 1255, 1990.

Wilson, F. A., & Neuhauser, D. *Health Services in the United States.* Cambridge, MA: Ballinger, 1976.

Chapter **6**

Principles of Health Planning

BASIC CONCEPTS OF HEALTH PLANNING

Herman Hilleboe, M.D., one of the primary developers of modern health-services planning, described it as follows (1967):

> Planning is an orderly process, put in writing, of:
> 1. defining the extent and characteristics of community health problems and identifying unmet needs,
> 2. assessing available and potential resources,
> 3. establishing priority goals (by matching needs and resources and considering alternatives and their consequences),
> 4. formulating the necessary administrative action to achieve program goals, and
> 5. relating results to goals by continuing evaluative studies.

Gottlieb stated three assumptions underlying health services planning:

- Resources are scarce; thus ways must be found to secure optimum value from allocations devoted to health.
- Health care serves social purposes and should therefore be valued above activity undertaken in pursuit of economic or other social ends.
- An effective health-care system is rooted in responsiveness to consumer needs and requires public accountability.

Another developer of modern health planning, Leonard Rosenfeld, summed up these thoughts well: "The aim of planning must be the achievement of optimum use of available resources for the betterment of human welfare." A contrasting, more contemporary view of the purposes of health planning, eschewing ethical considerations, was described by Marmor and Bridges: "There is a common impetus to health planning in the United States and other industrial countries: the concern to curb rapidly escalating costs."

Health-services planning occurs on two levels: macro and micro. The macro level is that of a health-services system, for the nation, a region, or one or more states. The micro level is that of an institution, such as a hospital or a health maintenance organization; a single, categorical health service provided to a geographic area, such as family planning or chronic-disease prevention; or a health-care provider's private office.

In their useful textbook and guide, *Basic Health Planning Methods*, Spiegel and Hyman describe six common types of health-services planning, all of which can take place at both the macro and micro levels (p. 11),:

- Problem solving planning: Identifying and resolving a specific problem, using the scientific method.
- Program planning: Setting a course of action to deal with a circumscribed problem, usually one that has already been described elsewhere.
- Coordination of efforts and activities planning: Aiming to increase the availability, efficiency, productivity, and effectiveness of various activities and programs.
- Planning for resource allocation: Choosing among various alternatives defined in earlier stages of the planning process in order to achieve the optimal outcome, given limited resources.
- Creation of a plan: Developing a blueprint for action, including recommendations and supporting data.
- Design of standard operating procedures: Creating sets of standards of practice and/or criteria for operation and evaluation.

One or more of these types of planning is part of any planning process.

GOALS AND OBJECTIVES

Regardless of the type of planning, to achieve success, it is essential that its desired goals and objectives be lucidly stated, understood, and agreed to by all parties concerned. The most frequent cause of failure in planning is neglecting to establish clear, agreed-upon goals and objectives, either as the first step or at least before the program-planning phase (step 4 in the Hilleboe formulation) is begun.

Goals are broad, usually long-range statements of ideal desired outcomes. For example: "All Americans shall have equal access to health care of high quality." Objectives refer to specific targets of action that are considered to be attainable. They are usually to be reached within a named time. The degree to which the program achieves its objective within the time specified should be measurable. For example: "Within 10 years there shall be one primary care practitioner for every 1,000 Americans." Clear definition of goals and objectives delineating and justifying the pathway being followed is essential for effective planning.

Obviously one cannot write a *complete* set of goals and objectives before beginning a planning process. In fact, at the beginning it is more likely that one can write goals rather than objectives. But as data are gathered—and no planning process can take place without data gathering—then specific objectives can be defined. As the planning process proceeds, it may be appropriate or necessary to add to or modify earlier goals and objectives. This "feedback-loop" mechanism is one of the principal engines of the planning process.

Realism is an essential element of any effective health-planning process and program. If the goals set are unrealistic (e.g., "Drug-free America" as the goal for the "Drug War," in a nation of 100 million users of alcohol and more than 50 million users of tobacco), the resultant program will often be incapable of achieving any positive results and may produce negative ones (as it does in the case of the "Drug War" [Nadelmann]).

Whatever health or health-care problem one is facing, to achieve a positive outcome, that problem must be realistically vulnerable to successful attack using the contemplated methods. Realism requires adequate data gathering and scientific (as contrasted with, say, ideological) interpretation of it. Realism permits sound priority setting (see Hilleboe, above). The establishment of useful and potentially effective goals and objectives is rooted in the latter.

Extrinsic and Intrinsic Goals and Objectives

The goals and objectives of the planning process are substantive. They define the desired physical and programmatic, functional *outcomes* of the planning process. They describe the reason the planning process of which they are a product was undertaken in the first place. They can be called *extrinsic*. Examples: What functions will the new or remodeled building serve? What is the new program for family planning intended to achieve? Why is the new program necessary?

One can also state goals and objectives *for* the planning process itself. These can be called *intrinsic*. They describe technical planning entities: what kind of product (a report, an analysis, a functional program, a building design, a construction schedule, a personnel recruitment and training program) is to be created by when. Intrinsic goals and objectives are used to measure the effectiveness of the planning process on its own terms: Were planning meetings held? How many? Who participated? Was a functional program developed? Did the physical plans provide for the spaces required to carry out the functional program? Was everything done on time? In planning, the term *goals and objectives* usually refers to extrinsic ones. That is the case in the balance of this chapter.

FAILURE TO DEFINE GOALS AND OBJECTIVES

When planners fail clearly to state usable goals and objectives (and this happens with depressing frequency in health-services planning in the United States), they usually encounter the following pitfalls:

- There is no way to evaluate the effectiveness of the planning process because what was being planned for was never defined.
- Reams of data are collected, much of them useless because of a lack of focus. (Without a statement of goals and objectives, data needs cannot be defined.)
- Inadequate data are collected, and decisions are made on the basis of incomplete knowledge and understanding.
- Ideology or preconceived notions, rather than science, is used to interpret the data.
- Planning for health-services *functions* and *operations* is confused with and sometimes superseded by planning for a *building*.

Several reasons account for the fact that development of goals and objectives is sometimes ignored in the planning process or that they are written so vaguely as to be meaningless and useless. First, the larger the group of interests affected by the proposed program, the more difficult it is to define goals and objectives that all parties can agree to. It is sometimes easier to skip this stage than go through the political process necessary to hammer them out.

Second, some of the parties involved may have goals and objectives they feel would not be (1) accepted under close scrutiny, (2) justified by data collection and analysis, or (3) economically feasible. If such persons are in positions of power from which they can develop and implement programs without setting written goals and objectives, they will often do so. Third, the glitter of the *techniques* of planning—the collection and analysis of data, the designing of administrative structures and staffing patterns, the development of budgets, and above all, the laying out of space—can easily outshine the fundamental, unglamorous, at times much more difficult job of determining "Why are we doing this?"

FUNCTION AND FORM

One outcome of much health-services planning activity is a new or remodeled building. In practice, it is impossible to design a building to meet specified health-services needs unless there is a *functional program*. The latter is a specification of activities, expected clientele, hours of service, staffing, organizational structure, projected budget, and so on. However, to develop a functional program, goals and objectives must be defined clearly. Buildings have been designed and built without a functional program.

Failure to define goals and objectives often leads planners to focus on the layout of the building rather than its intended function. The blueprints show rooms and corridors, doors and windows, closets and conference rooms. But nowhere is there a document, the functional program, showing how these spaces are to be used once they become a reality in concrete and steel. In this case, the tendency is to design the building to fit the available land and/or to spend the available money.

Building to occupy available land or spend available money rather than to meet defined needs by achieving specified goals and objectives of course violates Frank Lloyd Wright's elemental architectural dictum: "Form should follow function." The question What spaces are required to meet these needs? should be asked at the beginning of the planning process. The question is never asked in this scenario. Rather, toward the end of it, often after construction has started, someone says, "What needs do we meet with this space?" Many concrete and steel disasters could have been avoided if the planners had followed the orderly process described by Dr. Hilleboe.

PLANNING AND VALUES

In setting goals and objectives, it is important to remember there is no such thing as "value free planning" (Fein). Every planner and participant in the planning process is influenced by her or his "ideological baggage." The latter influences, indeed determines, one's value judgements and ordering of social priorities. Recall Rosenfeld's statement on the aim of planning: "It must be the achievement of *optimum use* of *available resources* for *the betterment of human welfare"* (emphasis added).

The very fact that Dr. Rosenfeld included "the betterment of human welfare" in his description of the aim reflects his personal values. The pecuniary approach to planning described by Marmor and Bridges reflects other values. Further, even within Dr. Rosenfeld's description, the definition of just what constitutes "optimum use," "available resources," and "the betterment of human welfare" will vary from person to person. Even in the presence of scientifically gathered data, each person's social values and priorities will strongly influence the nature of the definitions.

The workings of the health-care system have many outcomes. Some serve the needs of the people receiving health services. Others serve the personal nonhealth needs of people who work within the system. Meeting these two sometimes disparate sets of needs requires establishing two sometimes disparate sets of goals and objectives. Often the goals and objectives of those who work in the health-care system are the same as those of the people being served, that is, improving health status and combating disease. On occasion, however, they are not.

Provider needs and goals can be of a different order than those of patients: power, profits, prestige, institutional preservation and growth, career advancement, intellectual stimulation and development, and political gain. If two sets of goals and objectives exist side by side, spelled out in writing or not, and if there are unresolved conflicts between them, the result often is irrational, or no, planning.

THE PLANNING PROCESS

The basic concepts of health-services planning are straightforward. The fragmented health-care system in the United States, however, affects the nature of the technical planning process (Tierney & Waters). The science of planning, as noted above, consists of collecting and using data. The type and quantity of data needed depend on the existing level of health knowledge and planning knowledge, the particular health-care component being planned for, and characteristics of the larger social framework in which it is found. When planning is done correctly, that is, as a continuous, cyclical whole (Sigmond), all categories of data are relevant throughout, although one may be more heavily relied upon at one stage than another.

Planning for health services requires data on (1) the population to be served; (2) its health status; and (3) existing health-care resources and their utilization.

Without such information, one cannot determine whether the expressed *demand* for health services is greater than, equal to, or less than the *need* for health services. (*Demand* is a measure of the quantity and quality of health-care services that consumers want. *Need* is the quantity and quality of health services that health professionals estimate are required, based on various epidemiological indices and health and disease status and health-services use.)

Without planning data, there is no baseline against which one can measure the impact of implemented programs. Information is needed on the extent to which anticipated changes in health status occur, at what cost, and with what positive or negative side effects. Indeed, baseline data provide the foundation for systems of continuous feedback, systems that must be in place if inappropriate goals or inadequate work activities are to be identified and corrected.

Measuring Health Status

The first step is to measure health and illness levels in the population to be served. This can be the population of the nation as a whole, a defined community, or users of an existing service that is a candidate for redesign. Then the health-service needs of the target population can be estimated.

Some illustrative demographic data is discussed in Chapter 3. A population's health status is assessed by measures of mortality and morbidity or combinations of the two. Traditionally, mortality—maternal, infant, perinatal, and other, age-adjusted death rates—has been the primary indicator. Mortality indexes, however, are less than optimal measures of health. Their interpretation is confounded by multiple causes of death, poor reporting systems, and the shift over time from acute to chronic diseases as the major killers. Furthermore, death is an opposite of health; it is only an indirect measure of health status.

Measures of morbidity (the presence of a disease condition or active pathology) and disability (restricted performance of normal roles) present similar problems of collection and interpretation as well as others. There are a limited number of reportable diseases, and selective reporting leads to inaccurate data (Blum, 1974). In addition, the definition and classification of morbidity states can be difficult. In ethnically different populations, the same clinically defined disease may be indicated by different complaints. A cross-culturally valid index for each disease would be useful, one encompassing physical, emotional, and social causal factors; incidence (the number of new cases in a specified time); prevalence (the total number of extant cases in a specified time); duration; and severity.

In the National Health Survey (see Appendix II), disability is measured by the number of days of restricted activity in the preceding six months. The survey gathers data from a random sample of civilian, noninstitutional households. In another survey, conducted by the Social Security Administration, respondents are classified along a continuum based on the extent of their work limitations. Although the resultant "functional limitation index" provides a greater degree of specificity about disability, highly sensitive measures of acute and chronic disability are still unavailable.

Planners also measure the health status of a population by its present level of service use, frequency, waiting times, who is and isn't using presently available services, and so forth. These data, also part of the description of existing resources, reflect demand rather than need, but they are useful.

Describing Existing Resources

The next step is to undertake an inventory and evaluation of existing services (Spiegel & Hyman). There are three kinds of resources to be described: human, physical, and financial. For personnel, the number, age, sex, education, specialization, type of practice, productivity, geographic location, and availability must be determined, along with the output of operating and approved training programs. Existing sources of care must be inventoried by number, distribution, and characteristics such as size, type, volume, and quality of services offered; physical condition; licensure and accreditation status; policies; financial solvency; and referral patterns.

For each facility, patient characteristics must be described and utilization measures such as number of patient visits, average daily census, percentage occupancy, and average length of stay compiled. Financial data concerning the number and types of insurance mechanisms, government-supported programs, median family income, and sources of philanthropy must be obtained.

Determining Unmet Needs

This is the central step of the program-planning process. The data on health status enable the planners to estimate total health-services needs. From the description of the existing resources and the data on health services use, the planners can then estimate the portion of total need that is being met by the existing resources. The balance of the need, what is not being covered, is called the unmet need. Available resources constitute the supply side of the planning equation; sociodemographic factors, health-status measures, and professional assessments of undetected problems make up the demand-need side. By using the available mathematical tools and subjective estimates, the planner weighs one against the other and both against established standards to identify problems requiring attention (Spiegel & Hyman).

Program Planning

The next stage of the planning process is creating a program to meet unmet needs. At this point, the original goals must be reconsidered in light of the data obtained and analyzed. Goals may remain unchanged or redefined, reduced, or enlarged in scope. Objectives can now be written with more specificity. For a successful outcome, the refining of goals and objectives after the unmet needs have been determined and before program planning begins is critical.

In planning a program to meet unmet needs, the following (similar to the description of existing resources) must be provided for: description of services to be offered; personnel requirements and staffing patterns; policy-setting and administrative structure and mechanisms; financing systems to raise, budget, and pay out the funds needed for program operation; physical space; and a means for program evaluation and ongoing forward planning. As mentioned earlier, in order to have the best chance of creating a service that will truly meet community needs, program planning should always precede space planning.

If at all possible, before implementation, proposed programs should be tested by one means or another. It is rarely possible in the real world to run a purely scientific prospective experiment of a planned program before it is fully implemented. However, it is often possible to undertake a retrospective evaluation of similar previously implemented programs. This can be done through the literature, by private mail and telephone surveys, and by direct observation. This kind of analysis, not always done in the real world, can prove very useful. Pitfalls can be skirted, reinvention of the wheel can be avoided, and successful planning and implementation strategies can be adapted to use.

Evaluation

Once implemented, programs should be evaluated. Are the goals and objectives being met? Is the program cost-effective? Are there defects which could and should be remedied? In terms that still apply, Taylor described a two-pronged approach: evaluation for administrative purposes (are targets being met within specified time frames and in accordance with standards set?) and evaluation for plan revision (are original goals appropriate, the necessary resources being developed as anticipated?). Blum outlined five levels of evaluation:

1. *Activity*. Is the program operative?
2. *Criteria*. Is the program operating according to standards (of quality, access, etc.)?
3. *Cost*. Are program costs in line with those agreed upon? Can unit cost be improved?
4. *Effectiveness*. How well is the program achieving the desired output?
5. *Outcome validity*. To what extent has the program realized the ultimate goal for which it was designed?

It is important to avoid biased measures of outcome. Indeed, the literature on laboratory and field experiments is replete with cautions against evaluator contamination. Program designers are advised against evaluating their own programs, evaluators against implementing their own recommendations. Evaluations can fail in two ways, one of them scientific. The evaluative methods can be inadequate or faulty; that is, one or more of the five elements of evaluation described by Blum can be missing or incorrectly done. The second failure is the inability to produce "acceptable" findings, that is, those consistent with the policymaker's commitment to program success. A planning imperative thus becomes clear: As part of the original planning process, a coalition of support for thorough and scientific program evaluation, one that will hold together regardless of political repercussions, must be formed.

AN EXAMPLE OF PLANNING: DEALING WITH HOSPITAL PROBLEMS

The Problems

There are many problems faced by the hospital sector (see Chapter 3) that could be solved or at least ameliorated with an effective planning process. (Note that this list is slightly different from the one given in Chapter 3. The foci of the two are slightly different.) One major problem the hospital system faces is costliness (see Chapter 7); a second is oversupply of beds; and a third the imbalance between acute and long-term care.

As noted previously, the problem of cost is made worse by the inadequate supply of long-term beds for patients who have recovered from the acute phase of their illness but are still plagued by its long-term outcomes and, in many cases, the complications of poorly managed old age. Freymann has pointed out that the imbalance did not develop by accident (pp. 47–48; first paragraph also quoted in Chapter 3):

> The mold from which today's health care system was cast took its shape around 1850. There were still relatively few general hospitals or health facilities of any type in Britain and the fledgling United States, but the institutional organization of health care was already firmly established. Separate administration and staffing of the curative services for acute, chronic, and psychiatric illnesses became such a strong precedent that it continues even when all three components have a common source of support, as they do now in Britain. . . .
>
> As the four disparate fragments of our system for delivering care developed (acute, long term, psychiatric, and preventive services), the voluntary hospital component was the only one whose primary institutional objective was always treatment of disease. Voluntary hospitals were able to cater to patients selected for certain illnesses, generally acute ones, because donors were entitled to prescribe the scope of their charity, and because a medical staff that contributed its time without remuneration could reasonably dictate the nature of its worth. Both the philanthropic trustees and the medical staffs agreed on leaving to the state the prevention of disease and the intractable problems of mental illness and chronic infirmity [as well as care for an increasing proportion of the poor and otherwise unable to pay].

Also pointed out in Chapter 3 were the difficulties created by vertically organized administrative structures not well integrated horizontally at the service levels and the isolation of many hospitals from the real health and medical needs of their communities. Referring to the latter, Freymann (p. 74) describes the present era as the Age of Darwin and Freud since "most of our woes now stem from two causes: either our genetic heritage or the buffeting of our environment or both." He says, however, that many health-care institutions, not just short-term hospitals, are still armed primarily to fight the wars of the era immediately past, that is, the Age of Pasteur when "infection was the main foe of medicine" (p. 13). This orientation arises not only from institutional rigidity but from the character of medical practice, which is still largely stuck in the Age of Pasteur as well, even though the bulk of the problems are those of the Age of Darwin and Freud.

Solutions

Rational planning can produce solutions to many of these problems. However, the planning process does not get started by itself. Nor, once started, does it have the internal equipment to maintain its rationality. Planning is done by people, not machines (although computers can be very helpful in the process). It is people who decide that there are problems, that they should be attended to, that rational planning can help attend to them, and that once under way, the planning process should be kept within the bounds of rationality. But these are all *political* decisions, not technical ones. It is important at all times to be aware of the ultimately political nature of the planning process and to be able to deal with it.

For example, the adoption of Freymann's "mission-oriented" hospital approach (see also Chapter 3) would go a long way toward solving or at least ameliorating many of the problems hospitals face. But its adoption would require a serious commitment to planning and to implementation. That is a political matter, not a technical one.

As noted previously, Freymann's mission-oriented hospital has two principal attributes: (1) each hospital has a mission defined and continuously modified by the specific needs of the community services; (2) individuality and flexibility are secured by ongoing use of a rational planning process (p. 248). The concept is based on four "theorems" (Freymann, pp. 247–248):

1. The need for medical cure that dominated people's minds from the dawn of time to the end of the Age of Pasteur will wane, but the need for total health care will remain.
2. Health care must be a continuum, because a healthy life is a continuum from conception to death, not a vacuum punctuated by episodes of illness.
3. Since the needs of each individual vary widely, an organization meeting these needs cannot be frozen into classification by organ, by diagnosis, or by medical specialty.
4. Since the mission of the health care system is to maintain health, the system should interfere as little as possible with the functional capacity of those it serves. Ambulatory or home care are ideals; confinement to an institution must be dictated only by biologic necessity.

As pointed out in Chapter 3, the mission-oriented approach would make the hospital into a health center rather than an illness center. Hospitals would relate to the needs of their communities in a rationally planned manner. Distinctions among acute, chronic, and preventive services would be discarded. The integration of acute and chronic services and the introduction of effective preventive services could make a major contribution to cost containment.

Problems and Planning

In 1980 Peter Rogatz, a respected observer of the hospital scene, predicted that the following changes would take place during the 1980s:

- The supply of hospital beds will decrease; the average hospital will increase in size; and hospitals increasingly will offer complex services.
- Regulation will become more, not less, a part of hospital life.
- Ambulatory surgery will become increasingly common.
- Home-care services will expand.
- Long-term facilities will increase, and special housing for the elderly will become more commonplace.
- Hospitals will become increasingly interested in and attached to health maintenance organizations.
- The hospice movement will expand.

His predictions have proved largely correct. However, the problems and changes have been dealt with in a haphazard, uneven, *unplanned* manner. A comprehensive health-planning system might well be able to make a real contribution to insuring that productive change takes place. But what is the key to that, and is it possible to find that key in the United States? In the past, there have been several national health-care planning programs in the United States.* However, virtually all vestiges of them were swept away by the Reagan administration, to which, it seemed, *planning* was a dirty word.

Thus, Dr. Kropf tells us (1990), as the United States entered the 1990s, the "Federal government provides massive sums of money to be used by state governments, private for-profit and not for-profit hospitals physicians and other professionals" and "does not, however, have a plan for what services should be provided with the money,

---

*For more detail on the history of health planning in the United States, see S. Jonas, "Planning for Health Services," pp. 390–403, in S. Jonas, ed., *Health Care Delivery in the United States*, 3rd ed. (New York: Springer Publishing Co., 1986), and R. Kropf, "Planning for Health Services," pp. 326–339, in A. Kovner, ed., *Health Care Delivery in the United States*, 4th ed. (New York: Springer Publishing Co., 1990).

how many hospitals should exist and where, or how many physicians should practice in various cities and states."

Planning and Payment

Rashi Fein, chairman of the Institute of Medicine's Committee on Health Planning Goals and Standards, said in his preface to the committee's report (Institute of Medicine, p. iii): "The committee believes that the forces at work in the American health care system, including the various reimbursement mechanisms, cannot be countered by a health planning effort that is divorced, among other limiting factors, from the flow of funds." The theme that in order to be effective, planning must be linked to payment for services is one that has long bedeviled the U.S. health-care system. At present there is virtually no health-services planning going on, whether linked to payment or not. Will that situation change?

Henrik Blum, a longtime analyst of health planning, had his doubts (1983):

> Can there be meaningful health planning when so little else is publicly planned? It is my conviction that how health planning is set up is not altogether a result of special interest forces. Its mandate is determined by such societal forces as traditions, socioeconomic political outlooks, formal governance structures, and availability of resources. A society such as ours has strong anticollective biases, fears of government expressed as endless built in checks and balances, many levels of government, and many regional differences. Thus we will surely require, but have a difficult time developing, a strong national sense of direction that is melded with powerful state if not local participation to allow for ample variation in accordance with local needs and yet falls within nationally set goals. Our planning machinery is likely to be set up in just those ways that have allowed the health sector to create the problems that upset us so. Only under truly stressful shortages of resources, major calamities, or war are major changes going to be demanded of a given sector. That is what we are seeing today, and the official health planning machinery continues very much to one side of the action.

In 1990 the situation is no different.

REFERENCES

Blum, H. L. *Planning for Health: Development and Application of Social Change Theory.* New York: Human Sciences Press, 1974.

Blum, H. L. *"Health Planning: Lessons for the Future,* by Bonnie Lefkowitz" (book review). *Inquiry, 20,* 390, 1983.

Fein, R. "Priorities and Decision Making in Health Planning." *Israel Journal of Medical Sciences, 10,* 67, 1974.

Freymann, J. G. *The American Health Care System: It Genesis and Trajectory.* New York: Medcom Press, 1974.

Gottlieb, S. "A Brief History of Health Planning in the United States." In *Regulating Health Facilities Construction,* ed. C. C. Havighurst. Washington, DC: American Institute for Public Policy Research, 1974.

Hilleboe, H. E. "Health Planning on a Community Basis." Ann Arbor, MI: Delta Omega Lecture, School of Public Health, University of Michigan, July 31, 1967 (mimeographed).

Institute of Medicine, Committee on Health Planning Goals and Standards. *Health Planning in the United States: Selected Policy Issues.* 2 Vols. Washington, DC: National Academy Press, 1981.

Kropf, R. "Planning for Health Services." In *Health Care Delivery in the United States,* ed. A. Kovner 4th ed. New York: Springer Publishing co., 1990.

Marmor, T. R., & A. Bridges. "American Health Planning and the Lessons of Comparative Policy Analysis." *Journal of Health Politics, Policy and Law, 5,* 419, 1980.

Nadelmann, E. "Drug Prohibition in the United States: Costs, Consequences, and Alternatives." *Science, 245,* 939, 1989.

Rogatz, P. "Directions of the Health System for the New Decade." *Hospitals,* January 1, 1980, p. 67.

Rosenfield, L. S. "Problems in Planning Community Health Services." *Bulletin of the New York Academy of Medicine, 44,* 164, 1968.

Sigmond, R. M. "Health Planning." *Milbank Memorial Fund Quarterly,* 46 (supp.), 91, 1968.

Spiegel, A. D., & H. H. Hyman. *Basic Health Planning Methods.* Germantown, MD: Aspen Systems, 1978.

Taylor, C. E. "Stages of the Planning Process." In *Health Planning: Qualitative Aspects and Quantitative Techniques,* ed. W. A. Reinke. Baltimore, MD: Johns Hopkins University Press, 1972.

Tierney, J. T., & W. J. Waters. "The Evolution of Health Planning." *The New England Journal of Medicine, 308,* 95, 1983.

Chapter 7

Financing and Cost Containment

INTRODUCTION

All the money for health care comes from the people. Most of it goes to pay the institutional and individual providers for their services. Third parties (a party other than the patient or provider, usually an insurance company) handling money transfers retain a certain percentage. Since the United States lacks a single national health-care payment mechanism covering everybody, just how the money gets from the people to the providers is a complicated matter. The first part of this chapter describes the health-care financing system. The second part examines certain aspects of the problem of rising costs and develops a comprehensive approach to deal with it.

In the first chapter we described the five major components of the health-care system: health-care institutions, personnel, "health commodities" firms, education research institutions, and the financing system. The latter makes it possible for the first four to interact with each other and to produce for the recipients of their services what we call health care.

One useful way to analyze the health-care financing system is to divide the analysis into four categories: how much money is spent, where the money comes from (direct out-of-pocket, private insurance, etc.), what it is spent on (fees to individual providers, hospital services, drugs, etc.), and how it is paid out to the providers (item-of-service, per unit of care, etc.).

HEALTH CARE FINANCING
How Much Is Spent

In 1988, health-care payments totaled about $540 billion, an increase
of 10.4 percent over the previous year (ONCE, p. 1).* The 1988 inflation rate was 4.1 percent (USBoC, Table 757). About 89 percent of
total expenditures went for personal health services. The balance
paid for research, facilities construction, program administration,
private health insurance administration, and public health services.
Health-care spending accounted for 11.1 percent of the gross national
product (GNP); that figure is almost 25 percent higher than the
percentage of GNP spent by the country with the next highest spending rate, Sweden, and over 30 percent higher than in Canada (USBoC,
Table 1444). Sweden has one of the most comprehensive national
health services in the world. Canada has a comprehensive national
health insurance (NHI) program that is being examined closely by
both proponents and opponents of NHI in this country (see Chapter
8).

In both absolute and relative terms, national health expenditures
have grown considerably over the years (see Table 7.1). Between 1960
and 1988, national health-care payments increased twentyfold. Per
capita health payments increased by almost 15 times. In contrast, the
GNP increased only by about 9.5 times. In 1960, health-care expenditures accounted for only 5.3 percent of the GNP. Between 1970
and 1985, the annual rate of increase in health-care expenditures was
constantly in the double-digit range, even when inflation and the
GNP growth rate were not. Why this happens is matter of much
cogitation and controversy. Many attempts have been made to put a
brake on health-care cost increases, none very successful. That may
be because a correct causal analysis has not been done. This is a
subject to which we return in the last section of this chapter.

Where the Money Comes From

As noted above, all the money for health services ultimately comes
from the people. The phrase "where the money comes from" really
means "who is collecting the money, and how do they do it?" There
are many variants. For example, direct government programs (the

---

*This section is based largely on the article "National Health Expenditures, 1988," by
the Office of National Cost Estimates, *Health Care Financing Review*, *11*(4) (Summer
1990), 1–54, abbreviated ONCE in the text.

Department of Veterans Affairs hospital system, state mental hospitals, local public general hospitals) are supported mainly by tax revenues. Charitable contributions provide the primary support for the voluntary agencies. Private providers are supported by several sources: direct pay by patients, government tax-supported programs (e.g., Medicaid, a welfare-based system that pays for some health services for the poor), government social insurance (e.g., Medicare, a part of the Social Security System that pays for some health services for persons 65 and over and certain others), private insurance (e.g., not-for-profit Blue Cross, or commercial for-profit, such as Metropolitan Life), and others.

Figure 7.1 shows that government provided more than 40 percent of the health-care dollar in 1988, 29.9 percent from the federal government, 10.7 percent from the state and local governments (ONCE, p. 1). Private health insurance covered about 29 percent of payments. (Interestingly, while benefits grew 11 percent between 1987 and 1988, premium income to the insurance companies grew almost 12 percent.) In 1988 direct out-of-pocket payments accounted for less than 24 percent of monies paid (see Figure 7.1). ("Third party payment" is a major feature of the U.S. health-care delivery system. For many patients, care is provided under a direct private [usually unwritten] contract between themselves and the provider of care. But that care is often *paid for* not by the patient directly but by a health insurance company, Medicare, Medicaid, or certain other sources, referred to as the third party.)

Total personal health-care expenditures, per capita amounts, and percentage distribution by source of funds for the major sources of funds in selected years from 1960 to 1988 are shown in Table 7.2. Figure 7.1 shows that out-of-pocket payments declined significantly between 1960 and 1988. During that period, the shares of government and private health insurance rose significantly.

Private Health Insurance

There are two kinds of private health insurance (ONCE, p. 17). Blue Cross–Blue Shield operates on a not-for-profit basis. Its surplus of income over expenditures does not go to shareholders; rather it goes back into the company in the form of expanded services and/or higher salaries for employees. The commercial companies (e.g., Metropolitan Life, Travelers, Aetna) operate on a for-profit basis. Some of their surplus of income over expenditures is paid to the owners of the company as profit.

TABLE 7.1 National health expenditures aggregate and per capita amounts, percent distribution, and average annual percent growth, by source of funds: Selected calendar years 1960–88

	1960	1965	1970	1975	1980	1985	1986	1987	1988
	Amount in billions								
National health expenditures	$27.1	$41.6	$74.4	$132.9	$249.1	$420.1	$450.5	$488.8	$539.9
Private	20.5	31.3	46.7	77.8	143.9	245.2	259.8	280.5	312.4
Public	6.7	10.3	27.7	55.1	105.2	174.9	190.7	208.3	227.5
Federal	2.9	4.8	17.7	36.4	72.0	123.4	132.8	144.0	157.8
State and local	3.7	5.5	9.9	18.7	33.2	51.5	57.9	64.3	69.6
	Number in millions								
U.S. population[a]	190.1	204.0	214.8	224.7	235.2	247.1	249.5	251.8	254.2
	Amount in billions								
Gross national product	$515	$705	$1,015	$1,598	$2,732	$4,015	$4,232	$4,524	$4,881
	Per capita amount								
National health expenditures	$143	$204	$346	$592	$1,059	$1,700	$1,806	$1,941	$2,124
Private	108	154	217	346	612	992	1,041	1,114	1,229
Public	35	50	129	245	447	708	765	827	895
Federal	15	24	83	162	306	500	532	572	621
State and local	20	27	46	83	141	208	232	256	274

Percent distribution

National health expenditures	100.0	100.0	100.0	100.0	100.0	100.0	100.0	100.0	100.0
Private	57.9	57.4	57.7	58.4	57.8	58.5	62.8	75.3	75.5
Public	42.1	42.6	42.3	41.6	42.2	41.5	37.2	24.7	24.5
Federal	29.2	29.5	29.5	29.4	28.9	27.4	23.9	11.6	10.7
State and local	12.9	13.2	12.9	12.2	13.3	14.1	13.3	13.2	13.8

Percent of gross national product

National health expenditures	11.1	10.8	10.6	10.5	9.1	8.3	7.3	5.9	5.3

Average annual percent growth from previous year shown

National health expenditures	10.4	8.5	7.2	11.0	13.4	12.3	12.3	8.9	—
Private	11.4	8.0	6.0	11.2	13.1	10.7	8.3	8.9	—
Public	9.2	9.2	9.1	10.7	13.8	14.8	21.9	9.1	—
Federal	9.6	8.4	7.6	11.4	14.6	15.5	29.8	10.6	—
State and local	8.2	11.1	12.5	9.2	12.1	13.5	12.6	7.9	—
U.S. population	0.9	1.0	1.0	1.0	0.9	0.9	1.0	1.4	—
Gross national product	7.9	6.9	5.4	8.0	11.3	9.5	7.6	6.5	—

a July 1 social security area population estimates.
Note: Numbers and percent may not add to totals because of rounding.
Source: Table 13, Office of National Cost Estimates, "National Health Expenditures, 1988," Health Care Financing Review, 11(4) (1990), 24.

Where it came from

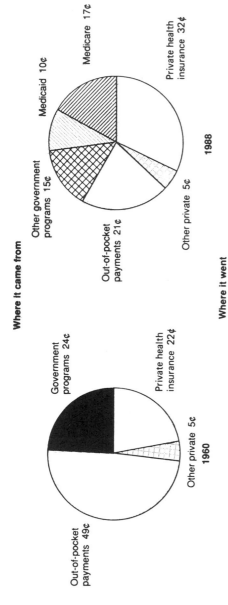

Government
programs 24¢

Private health
insurance 22¢

Other private 5¢

1960

Out-of-pocket
payments 49¢

Other government
programs 15¢

Medicaid 10¢

Medicare 17¢

Private health
insurance 32¢

1988

Other private 5¢

Out-of-pocket
payments 21¢

Where it went

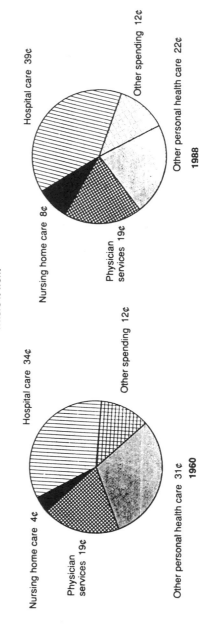

Hospital care 34¢

Other spending 12¢

Nursing home care 4¢

Physician
services 19¢

Other personal health care 31¢

1960

Hospital care 39¢

Other spending 12¢

Other personal health care 22¢

1988

Nursing home care 8¢

Physician
services 19¢

FIGURE 7.1 The nation's health dollar: 1960 and 1988

Source: Office of National Cost Estimates, "National Health Expenditures, 1988,"
Health Care Financing Review, 11(4), Figure 2, p. 3.

Private health insurance paid for about one-third of all personal health services in 1988. About 80 percent of private health insurance is provided by employers for workers and their families. It should come as no surprise, therefore, that the services for which the most insurance coverage is available are those used most heavily by the working population. For example, private insurance covered over 35 percent of hospital costs, 48 percent of physician services, and 42 percent of dental services but only 7 percent of home care and 1 percent of nursing-home costs (ONCE, p. 17). About 75 percent of Americans have some kind of private health insurance coverage. About 90 percent of them are under 65.

Out-of-Pocket Payments

Out-of-pocket payments include direct pay to providers for noninsured services, extra payments to providers of insurance-covered services who bill at an amount higher than the insurance company pays, and "deductibles" and "coinsurance" on health insurance benefits (ONCE, p. 18). A deductible is a flat amount, say $100 per individual or $250 per family, that a health-care beneficiary must pay out of pocket before insurance coverage begins for any health services received during some time period (usually a calendar year).

Coinsurance is a share, say 20 percent, of the payment for each service covered by insurance for which the beneficiary is responsible. The extra charges that some providers levy over what insurance pays are in addition to the coinsurance. Reflecting the different levels of third-party coverage for different health services, while out-of-pocket payments accounted for only 5.3 percent of hospital costs in 1988, they accounted for over 70 percent of the costs of medications.

Government Spending

Government spending has accounted for an increasing proportion of the health-care dollar since 1960. In that year, five years before Congress enacted Medicare, government's share was about 25 percent. By the early 1970s, it was about 40 percent. It has stayed in that range ever since (42.7 percent in 1988). Government covered about 5 percent of hospital costs and almost 49 percent of nursing-home costs in 1988 (ONCE, pp. 19–24). Together, Medicare and Medicaid covered about 30 percent of personal health-care costs in that year.

TABLE 7.2 Personal Health-care Expenditures Aggregate and Per Capita Amounts and Percent Distribution, by Source of Funds: Selected Calendar Years 1960–88

| | Total | Out-of-pocket payments | Third-party payments | | | Government | | | Medicare[a] | Medicaid[b] |
			Total	Private health insurance	Other private funds	Total	Federal	State and local		
					Amount in billions					
1960	$23.9	$13.3	$10.5	$5.0	$0.4	$5.1	$2.1	$3.0	—	—
1965	35.6	19.0	16.6	8.7	0.7	7.3	3.0	4.3	—	—
1970	64.9	25.6	39.3	15.2	1.7	22.4	14.6	7.8	$7.2	$5.1
1975	116.6	38.5	78.0	29.9	2.9	45.3	31.0	14.4	15.7	12.9
1980	218.3	58.4	159.9	65.3	7.6	87.1	63.5	23.6	36.4	24.8
1985	367.2	91.7	275.5	114.1	12.9	148.5	111.6	36.9	70.1	39.7
1986	397.7	96.8	300.9	125.3	13.5	162.1	120.5	41.6	75.4	42.9
1987	434.7	102.4	332.3	139.8	14.7	177.8	130.9	46.9	81.7	48.2
1988	478.3	113.2	365.1	155.2	15.9	194.0	143.2	50.8	89.7	52.3
					Per capita amount					
1960	$126	$70	$55	$26	$2	$27	$11	$16	—	—
1965	175	93	81	42	3	36	15	21	—	—
1970	302	119	183	71	8	104	68	36	(c)	(c)

Year										
1975	519	172	347	133	13	202	138	64	(c)	(c)
1980	928	248	680	277	32	370	270	100	(c)	(c)
1985	1,486	371	1,115	462	52	601	452	149	(c)	(c)
1986	1,594	388	1,206	502	54	650	483	167	(c)	(c)
1987	1,726	407	1,319	555	58	706	520	186	(c)	(c)
1988	1,882	445	1,436	610	63	763	564	200	(c)	(c)

Percent distribution

Year										
1960	100.0	55.9	44.1	21.0	1.7	21.4	8.9	12.5	—	—
1965	100.0	53.4	46.6	24.3	1.9	20.4	8.3	12.0	—	—
1970	100.0	39.5	60.5	23.4	2.6	34.6	22.6	12.0	11.1	7.8
1975	100.0	33.1	66.9	25.6	2.5	38.9	26.6	12.3	13.4	11.1
1980	100.0	26.8	73.2	29.9	3.5	39.9	29.1	10.8	16.7	11.4
1985	100.0	25.0	75.0	31.1	3.5	40.4	30.4	10.0	19.1	10.8
1986	100.0	24.3	75.7	31.5	3.4	40.8	30.3	10.5	19.0	10.8
1987	100.0	23.6	76.4	32.2	3.4	40.9	30.1	10.8	18.8	11.1
1988	100.0	23.7	76.3	32.4	3.3	40.6	29.9	10.6	18.8	10.9

aSubset of Federal funds.
bSubset of Federal and State and local funds.
cCalculation of per capita estimates is inappropriate.
NOTES: Per capita amounts based on July 1 social security area population estimates. Numbers and percents may not add to totals because of rounding.
Source: Office of National Cost Estimates, "National Health Expenditures, 1988," Health Care Financing Review, 11(4), (1990), Table 16, p. 31.

Medicare

The Medicare program was created by Title XVIII of the Social Security Act (ONCE, pp. 19–22). The legislation was passed by Congress in 1965 as part of President Lyndon Johnson's "Great Society" program. Originally, it provided payment for some health services for person 65 and older. In 1972 its coverage was broadened to include permanently disabled workers and their dependents who were eligible for old age, survivors, and disability insurance under Social Security, and persons with end-stage renal disease. There are two parts of Medicare: hospital insurance (HI), which also covers hospice and home health care, and supplementary medical insurance (SMI), which covers physician services, hospital outpatient care, and certain other services.

In 1988, Congress tried to expand Medicare by adding payment for extremely expensive hospital care ("catastrophic care"), pharmaceutical drugs, and certain other items. However, the cost was to be borne entirely by the elderly, especially the better-off elderly, and their protests led to the repeal of those provisions.

Medicare HI is funded primarily from Social Security taxes; SMI is funded primarily from general revenues. In 1988, Medicare payments, almost $86 million, accounted for about 8 percent of the total federal budget, up from 6 percent in 1980. In 1988, Medicare covered about 30 million persons 65 and over and more than 3 million disabled persons.

While Congress has enacted various cost-containment measures under Medicare, none have been very effective—for example, in the period 1984–1988 a cap on Medicare physician fees and a voluntary program to protect patients against being billed for more than Medicare would pay (called balance billing). During this time, spending for physician services grew twice as fast as that for hospital care. In the late 1980s a new fee schedule, the resource-based relative value scale (RBRVS), was developed. It is designed to bring down payments for procedure-based care such as surgery and raise payments for nonprocedure-based services like most primary care. In the early 1990s, it is gradually being implemented. Its impact will be closely followed.

Medicaid

In 1965 Congress also created Medicaid (sometimes also referred to as Title XIX of the Social Security Act [ONCE, pp. 22–23]). It is a welfare-based program that provides some coverage for some health services for some of the poor. It is supported by federal and state tax funds and administered by the states. Each state program is distinct from that of all the others; benefits and who is covered vary widely from state to state.

Title XIX requires the state to provide a set of 21 services to be eligible to receive federal funds for its program and stipulates that persons eligible for cash payments under the Supplementary Security Income program covering the aged, blind, and disabled, or Aid to Families with Dependent Children (usually, "welfare") be covered by Medicaid. However, each state decides who is to be covered by Welfare and what fees are to be paid to providers.

A combination of low-income eligibility requirements for welfare and low fees for providers (many of whom thus choose not to participate) leads to very limited coverage in many states. On the reverse side of the coin, a few of the wealthier states provide Medicaid coverage for the "medically indigent," persons in an income range deemed not low enough to qualify for welfare but low enough to make paying for health services a heavy burden.

In 1988, Medicaid covered about 11 percent of all personal health-care spending. About 23 million people received some kind of Medicaid coverage, but for many that care was far from comprehensive. Medicaid paid for about 45 percent of all nursing-home care.

Other Government Programs

Among other major government health programs are (ONCE, pp. 23–24) at the federal level, the Department of Defense, the Department of Veterans Affairs, and the Public Health Service including the National Institutes of Health (the Federal government's major biomedical research arm); at the state level, the state public health and mental hospital services; and at the local level, the local public general hospitals and local public health activities (see Chapter 5). These are paid for by tax funds. Together, they consume a relatively small proportion of the national health-care budget; for example, in 1988 national expenditures on public health services accounted for less than 3 percent of the total. By way of comparison, payments for program administration and the net cost of private insurance (administration and profit) together were about 65 percent higher than expenditures for public health services.

Where the Money Goes

Figure 7.1 shows that the shares of the physicians and "other spending" were the same in 1960 and 1988. During that period, the shares accruing to hospitals and nursing homes went up while that for "other personal health care" went down. Table 7.3 shows the

TABLE 7.3 National Health Expenditures, by Source of Funds and Type of Expenditure: Selected Calendar Years 1960–88

	Total	All private funds	Private Consumer Total	Private Consumer Out of pocket	Private Consumer Private insurance	Private Other	Government Total	Government Federal	Government State and local
					Amount in billions				
1988									
National health expenditures	$539.9	$312.4	$288.1	$113.2	$174.9	$24.3	$227.5	$157.8	$69.6
Health services and supplies	520.5	304.6	288.1	113.2	174.9	16.5	215.9	149.0	66.9
Personal health care	478.3	284.3	268.4	113.2	155.2	15.9	194.0	143.2	50.8
Hospital care	211.8	96.6	86.3	11.3	75.0	10.3	115.2	86.7	28.5
Physician services	105.1	70.0	69.9	19.9	50.0	0.0	35.2	28.7	6.4
Dental services	29.4	28.7	28.7	16.3	12.4	—	0.7	0.4	0.3
Other professional services	22.5	18.0	15.4	7.1	8.3	2.6	4.5	3.4	1.0
Home health care	4.4	1.1	0.8	0.5	0.3	0.3	3.3	2.6	0.7
Drugs and other medical nondurables	41.9	37.3	37.3	29.6	7.7	—	4.6	2.2	2.4

Vision products and other medical durables	10.8	3.6	8.6	7.6	1.0	—	2.3	2.0	0.2
Nursing home care	43.1	22.1	21.3	20.8	0.5	0.8	20.9	12.5	8.4
Other personal health care	9.3	1.9	—	—	—	1.9	7.4	4.7	2.7
Program administration and net cost of private health insurance	26.3	20.3	19.7	—	19.7	0.5	6.1	3.9	2.2
Government public health activities	15.9	—	—	—	—	—	15.9	1.9	14.0
Research and construction	19.4	7.8	—	—	—	7.8	11.5	8.8	2.7
Research	9.9	0.7	—	—	—	0.7	9.1	7.9	1.2
Construction	9.5	7.1	—	—	—	7.1	2.4	0.9	1.5

NOTES: — denotes less than $50 million. Research and development expenditures of drug companies and other manufacturers and providers of medical equipment and supplies are excluded from "research expenditures," but are included in the expenditure class in which the product falls. Numbers may not add to totals because of rounding.

Source: Office of National Cost Estimates, "National Health Expenditures, 1988," *Health Care Financing Review, 11*(4), (1990), Table 15, p. 30.

amounts paid for the several major categories of health care and other services as well as the sources of those payments by type of payor. Spending for health services and supplies accounted for 96 percent of total expenditures in 1988. Personal health care "includes services received by individuals in hospitals, nursing homes, office of physicians, dentists, and other licensed health professionals; home health care; drugs, vision care products, other durable and nondurable medical products," and that old standby, "miscellaneous" (ONCE, p. 4).

In 1988, 44 percent of all personal health-care spending went to hospitals, falling from a peak of 48 percent in 1982. Hospital payments cover inpatient and outpatient (clinic and emergency room) costs, including such items as capital costs; food; utilities; salaries for administrative, nursing, dietary, maintenance, technology, and other staff; the nonpayroll costs of laboratory and radiology services; physician fees billed through the hospital (e.g., for resident house staff, pathologists, and anesthesiologists); and medications.

Along with physicians (both allopathic, M.D.'s, and osteopathic, D.O.'s) and dentists, there are other categories of health-care providers who may be paid directly by the patient or the patient's insurer. Payments to them are counted in the "other professional services" category. Other health professionals who receive direct payments include psychotherapists (with a Ph.D. or other doctorate, a master's degree, and in some states no degree), chiropractors, podiatrists (foot care), speech pathologists and audiologists, optometrists (vision testing) and opticians (who make glasses), and in certain states physical therapists, acupuncturists, naturopaths, homeopaths, and other healers. The "other professional services" category also includes nonhospital outpatient agencies such as kidney dialysis centers, rehabilitation centers, and alcohol- and drug-treatment centers, certain types of HMO, and the community health centers.

Grouped together under "other spending" are home health care (preventive, supportive, therapeutic, and rehabilitative); drugs and other medical nondurables (such as bandages); vision products and other medical durables (hearing aids, braces, and wheelchairs); nursing-home care; government public health activities; and the old reliable, "all other."

How the Money Is Paid Out

Money is paid for health care by one of four modes: fee-for-service, unit of care, episode of care, and global budgeting. The predominant mode for paying physicians, dentists, and the private providers in the "other professional services" category above is fee-for-service. This piecework system is the oldest form of payment for health services. According to some (Jonas, 1978, pp. 319–326; Roemer), it is a major cause of many problems in the health-care system. It should be noted that the majority of people working in the health-care system— nurses, administrators, and other institutional staff; some physicians, dentists, and "other health professionals—are paid by salary.

Unit of care is a method for paying institutions by a unit of time, or a service such as use of the operating room or the provision of a laboratory test. "Per diem" (by the day) reimbursement for hospital or nursing-home care is a common form of unit-of-care payment. One method of paying physicians is unit of care—"capitation." The physician receives a flat rate for providing all medical care to a given patient for a designated period, usually a year. Only a small minority of U.S. physicians are paid by this method.

Episode of care is the method used in the diagnosis-related group (DRG) system of paying hospitals under Medicare. The hospital receives a flat rate for providing all the care required for a given diagnosis. The payment covers bed days, lab tests, X-rays, operations, and so forth, regardless of the actual volume of services used.

Under global budgeting, an institution or program receives a lump sum from its sponsoring authority to provide all services to all comers for a given time, usually a year. This is the common way of paying for VA hospitals, state mental hospitals, and local health departments. These institutions in turn may collect reimbursement from various insurance programs, government and private, for patients who have coverage. Monies collected in this manner usually go back to the sponsoring agency to offset the globally budgeted sum.

THE RISING COSTS OF HEALTH CARE

As noted above, health-care costs have been rising faster than the inflation rate since at least 1960, and the U.S. spends more of its GNP on health services than any other country in the world.* For many of

---

*This section is largely drawn from a paper by Steven Jonas, M. D., M.P.H., "Strengths and Limitations of the New Federalism: Regional Diversity and Financing," delivered on May 22, 1990, at the conference "Health Policy in the 21st Century: Global Issues, National Priorities, State and Local Solutions," sponsored by the Center for Health Policy of George Mason University, held in Arlington, VA. For an in-depth view of the problem, see Kenneth Thorpe, "Health Care Cost Containment," ed. in *Health Care Delivery in the United States*, 4th ed., ed. A. R. Kovner (New York: Springer Publishing Co., 1990).

the years since 1970, the rise in costs exceeded the rise of consumer price index by 100–200 percent (ONCE, Table 13; USBoC, Table 757). Since 1985, the former has outstripped the latter by a factor ranging from 2.4 to almost 4.

Nevertheless, the United States trails many of the world's industrial nations on such health indicators as life expectancy and infant mortality rate (USBoC, Table 1440). In 1988, life expectancy in the United States actually decreased compared with that in 1987, the first time that has occurred since World War II *(MVSR)*. This was apparently due to deficits in the quantity and quality of services provided to blacks for diseases that are preventable to a significant degree (Schwartz et al.). Furthermore, despite rising costs, or perhaps because of them, a significant proportion of the population has no health insurance coverage. In 1987, close to 33 million people, almost 14 percent of the population, were in that category (USBoC, Table 152). The health of significant portions of the black population in particular was declining sharply (Rosenthal).

Many words have been written about the problem of rising costs. The question why what we spend provides neither the world's highest health levels nor coverage for everyone has frequently been asked. Many interventions have been developed in the attempt to deal with the problem. None have been very effective.

The balance of this chapter is devoted to a discussion of the "cost-containment" problem from a perspective somewhat different from the usual one. It is based on the following premises:

- The reason the various interventions have generally failed is that they have not been aimed at the substantive (as contrasted with the formalistic) causes of the problem. (The word *substantive* in this context concerns who is doing what to whom, in what places, focusing on which health-disease problems, at what cost, the money being paid out in what way, and what health-disease problems are *not* being dealt with and why.)
- Nothing effective can be done in cost containment until the substantive causes of the problem are identified and addressed.
- It is unlikely that the substantive causes of ever-rising costs can be effectively addressed in the absence of comprehensive health-care reform, which also addresses the other major problems of the system (see also Chapter 8).

Previous Attempts to Contain Costs

Many of the attempts at cost containment have focused simply on the dollars paid in; that is, "supply-side" approaches:

- Freezing all health-care prices. (This occurred during the Nixon presidency; prices exploded after the freeze was lifted.)
- Capping hospital expenditures on a voluntary basis. (This occurred during the Carter presidency after the president had tried and failed to get Congress to pass a mandatory cap. One can imagine how well that approach worked.)
- Changing from a unit-of-care payment system (*per diem* rates) for hospitals to an episode-of-care system (DRGs). (This change occurred during the Reagan presidency. The gap between the health-care cost and the overall inflation rates was never higher.)

None of these attempts have been based on an analysis of the substantive *causes* of rising costs that might be found in the system itself. As all supply-side analyses do, they assumed it was simply the amount of dollars flowing in that determined prices. It appears that this is not the case. The alternative is to begin with an analysis of the system's problems. This approach is based on the concept that it is what the system does and does not do to and for patients and others that is the major driver of costs, not simply how many dollars are paid into it.

The Problem List

It is both depressing and instructive to observe that the United States is not much further along in dealing with its health-care problems than it was in 1932. The opening of the *Final Report* of the Committee on the Costs of Medical Care (1932) is quoted above in Chapter 1. Unfortunately, its terms still apply. To bring the CCMC's list up to date, almost 60 years later, one need only add that:

1. Costs are astronomical and routinely outstrip the general inflation rate.
2. Nowhere near what could be done in health promotion–disease prevention is done.
3. Medical labor is poorly distributed by specialty and geography; there is an inefficient, ineffective distribution of labor between the several health professions-occupations.
4. Institutional care is neither organized nor used in an effective manner.
5. The high-tech tail is wagging the health-care dog.
6. The deficiencies in primary care, already identified in the CCMC era when 90 percent of physicians were general practitioners (AAMC, 1932, pp. 23–24, 114–119) have worsened significantly.

7. Deficiencies in doctor-patient communication are significant and a major concern of patients.

In the late 1980s, there were many proposals on the table intending to "do something" about solving the problems from such disparate groups as the Committee on Labor and Human Resources (pp. 3–4), the National Association of Manufacturers (pp. 1–3), the Heritage Foundation (pp. v–vi), the National Leadership Commission on Health Care (pp. 1–23), the Oil, Chemical and Atomic Workers (pp. 1–5), the Committee for National Health Insurance (pp. 1–3), and the American Medical Association (see also Chapter 8).

The problem lists found in each of these documents are familiar. And it is interesting to note that allowing for some differences in emphasis related to the background and political-economic interests of their authors, the lists are remarkably similar. But these reports are also similar in what they generally do and do not do, having assembled the problem lists: They do not engage in much causal analysis.

They do not deal with the *substance* of the system and its problems. Why do we have these problems? What are their origins? Why have we not been able to solve them in 60 years? What is it in the system that drives costs ever higher? Just what does the system do and not do to and for patients? Who in the system is doing what and why? How do those activities contribute to and/or ameliorate the identified problems? For example, what is the role of the emphasis on hospital-based acute care in driving costs higher? Could a major increase in the provision of health-promotion–disease-prevention services in the ambulatory setting not only improve health but also save money? If yes, what has to be done substantively in the system to achieve that goal? Where does the resistance to change lie? Why do those who resist change resist change? What could be done to overcome the resistance?

Form and Substance

Failing to undertake *substantive* analysis, each organization above has come up with some *formalistic* solutions for dealing with the problems on their list. Subscribed to by one or more of these organizations are expand Medicare, eliminate Medicare, expand Medicaid, eliminate Medicaid, require all employers to cover their workers, substitute comprehensive coverage for the total population for employment-based coverage, expand catastrophic coverage, expand long-term coverage, set up some kind of national health service, establish a single (monopsony) payor system, maintain a multiple-payor system, establish fee schedules, eliminate deductibles and coinsurance, expand deductibles and coinsurance, cap hospital reimbursement, expand DRGs, eliminate DRGs, set up global budgets, separate capital-construction budgets, create consumer-generated competition, create provider-generated competition, eliminate tax deductibility for employer-paid health insurance premiums, strengthen planning mechanisms, eliminate any vestiges of health-systems planning, and so on.

As we can see, most of these recommendations deal with structural, formalistic matters, not substantive ones. Most of them have little relationship to identifiable causes of the problems. And many of those problems have a direct bearing on rising costs. For example, it is not Medicare per se that drives costs upward but how the Medicare benefit package (which favors acute hospital care) and the physician payment method (which until the mid-1980s paid "usual and customary fees") influenced the *substance* of the system: the type, quantity, and cost of the care. Furthermore, it should now be clear that it is impossible to deal with the problem of rising costs in isolation. The other problems on the list must also be dealt with.

That exercise involves some pain. It requires examining an institution that many feel uncomfortable or intimidated in examining, for personal, psychological, and political reasons. That exercise, looking for substantive causes, requires looking at the structure and function of the medical profession.

Examining Causes

If our car isn't running right, we don't usually deal with that problem by examining the design of the body and evaluating the comfort of the seats. We go to where the trouble is likely to be: the engine. If it is necessary to fix the engine to make the car run properly, that must be done, whether the task is hard or easy; otherwise, the car will continue not to run right. For better or worse, the engine of the U.S. health-care system is the medical profession. Health-care problem solvers must turn their attention to it.

Current Examinations: Scratching the Surface

Let us look more closely at a standard problem list with the customarily proposed solutions for each element. When they are assigned at all, the commonly attributed causes and suggested solutions are formalistic.

1. Problem: continually rising costs. Formalistic cause: continually expanding money supply coming into the system. Solution: Curtail the money supply.

2. Problem: inequity; the undersupply of health care to certain Americans due to the presence of financial barriers. Formalistic cause: a "lack of fairness." Solution: Create fairness by providing access for everyone to the present system of medical care.

3. Problem: deficiencies in the quality of care. Formalistic cause: The system for assuring quality leaves much to be desired. Solution: Make the quality-assurance system better.

4. Problem: oversupply of care in some cases. Formalistic cause: inadequate "utilization controls." Solution: Improve utilization controls.

5. Problem: the ever-increasing focus on acute-care, high-tech medicine. (This produces the ever-increasing focus on the high-tech preservation of fragile biological life at both ends of the age range. This focus gives little consideration to quality of life factors, or investment in methods which could improve the quality of life without expensive high-tech interventions.) Formalistic cause: the "technological imperative." Solution: There is none; this is a problem we just have to learn to live with (Ginzburg).

6. Problem: the malorganization of the health-care institutional sector. Formalistic cause: poor planning or the absence of effective free-market influences. Solution: Fix the planning system, or let the free market rip.

7. Problem: deficient primary care. Formalistic cause: not enough financial support for primary-care training in medicine. Solution: Provide some additional funds for primary care training. Alternatively, specify a certain number of publicly funded residency training slots for primary care.

8. Problem: the continued presence of the "preventable physical pain and mental anguish" referred to by the CCMC. (Since we know so much more about prevention than we used to, this problem has intensified over the years. For example, we know how to prevent or diminish the occurrence or impact of unwanted pregnancies, abortion, low-birthweight babies, prematurity, [and thus mental retardation]; and at the other end of the age range, heart disease, certain cancers, chronic lung disease, stroke, hypertension, debilitation and low-quality long life; and in between, sexually transmitted disease, intentional and unintentional personal-injury disability and death among other diseases and conditions [USPHS].) Formalistic cause: Most policymakers pay little attention to this one. Those who do usually refer to lack of reimbursement for preventive services as the

principal cause of the problem (Davis et al.). This leads to the conclusion that the provision of reimbursement is the solution.

9. Problem: Doctor-patient communication is deficient. Formalistic cause: As with the deficits in prevention, most policymakers pay little attention to this one. And as with prevention, those who do usually refer to lack of reimbursement for effective communication and recommend provision of such payment as the solution.

Delving Deeper

Some of the proposed solutions have been tried, without much success. For example, at one time or another we have curtailed the money supply, expanded coverage, contracted coverage, changed the reimbursement system, tried to monitor quality better, controlled utilization, planned or not planned. Why do these formalistic solutions, so reasonable on paper, not work? Perhaps because, to borrow a phrase from the medical scientist-writer Lewis Thomas, they are "half-way technologies." They don't get at the substantive causes of the problems.

The Medical Profession: the Engine of the System

The medical profession is at the center of the health-care system, whether that is a desirable state of affairs or not. It is the system's engine. Furthermore, to extend the analogy, it is an engine that happens to have much control over the steering wheel. Without the profession, the system cannot go anywhere. And when it goes, the direction that it takes is largely determined by the engine, not the owner of the vehicle, which happens to be the people of the United States.

There are four principal reasons accounting for this state of affairs (Jonas, 1988). First, the medical-licensing system gives physicians control over the central clinical functions of the health-care system: making diagnoses, performing surgery, and prescribing medications from a restricted list. Second, because of the special nature of the health-care market, physicians are the primary determinants of about two-thirds of the system's expenditures (Dyckman; Fuchs & Kramer). Third, among all health-care providers, physicians have the highest level of training in biomedical science, which provides the scientific basis for most health services. Fourth, for many people, the physician still has the role of healer, which for some assumes mystical proportions.

The view that the medical profession is central to the system and bears major responsibility for some of its major problems is supported by Dr. Leighton Cluff, former president of the Robert Wood Johnson Foundation. In "A Challenge to America's Physicians," which appeared in the Foundation's *1989 Annual Report*, Dr. Cluff considered this issue at some length.

Physicians in 1990 have a choice: either help address the problems facing the nation's health care system, or reject this obligation and let others make the attempt. . . . The twin obligations of medicine to serve individuals and society have drifted apart. Some way must be found to make these issues concordant. The issues seem obvious enough to everyone else: at the community, state, regional and national levels, people are alarmed. Too many physicians, it seems, are fiddling their familiar tune while the edifices of medicine are set ablaze by outsiders. . . .

There are no simple or easy solutions to the problems outlined earlier, and physicians cannot resolve them alone. Still, appropriate action that protects the best of what the nation has in personal medical care cannot occur without the collective involvement of physicians. For example:

- Physician choices about how they practice medicine account for a majority of health care expenditures and contribute significantly to rising health care costs;
- The increasing number of highly specialized physicians and medical services in suburban settings, contrasted with the unavailability of personal medical services in many rural and inner-city areas, depends very much on physicians' personal and career choices;
- Unnecessary duplication of medical services in hospitals and by physicians in communities and regions is significantly influenced by doctors;
- The fragmentation of medical services—which often requires patients to become their own diagnosticians and to seek care from multiple, non-integrated providers—could be largely remedied by physician leadership;
- Disparities in the use of technology and medical procedures between regions and hospitals can be addressed by physicians enlarging their concentration on the care of individuals to include the impact of how their actions affect the community;
- Inequity in access to personal medical services, although it has many roots and although many physicians conscientiously try to provide services to people in need, has not been addressed adequately by physicians as a group; and
- The nation's health care problems are changing: the rise in chronic health problems and AIDS, the demands of alcohol and drug abuse, the problems of mental illness, the toll of violence—all call for physicians to take the forefront in amelioration efforts.

It is clear from this analysis that if we are to correct the defects of the system, we must determine what's wrong with the engine. We must find out *why* it doesn't take us where we want to go. We must be prepared to repair it or even to change its design (hopefully in a way that will maintain professional control of professional functioning). Dr. Cluff makes the point that if the medical profession does not do a better of job of steering, some outside agency is going to come along and take control of that function completely.

This analysis is a metaphor for saying that to find the *causes* of many of the problems of the health-care system, we must look at the medical profession and how it functions. Once we do that causal analysis, we can make substantive rather than formalistic changes in the system, and we will thus seriously address its problems.

The Problem List Revisited

As a first approximation of that effort, let us return to the list of problems, supposed causes, and recommended solutions presented above. Then, putting the understanding of the physician as the engine into the analysis, let us consider some different recommendations for each stated problem.

1. Problem: continually rising costs. Usual cause: continually expanding money supply coming into the system. Usual solution: Curtail the money supply.

Medical-practice-based cause: piecework (fee-for-service) system for paying physicians with resultant high-income possibilities-expectations. Alternative solution: Gradually change that system to the one used for the majority of health-care workers—salary.

2. Problem: inequity, the undersupply of health care to certain Americans due to the presence of financial barriers to care. Usual cause: a "lack of fairness." Usual solution: Create fairness by providing access for everyone to the present system of medical care.

Medical-practice-based cause: Financial barriers are created at least in part by the private entrepreneurial nature of much medical practice. Alternative solution: Gradually phase out that system.

3. Problem: deficiencies in the quality of care. Formalistic cause: The system for assuring quality leaves much to be desired. Solution: Make the quality-assurance system better.

Medical-practice-based cause: Physicians are not trained to keep effective track of the quality of their care. Neither are they trained to work collegially to maintain uniformly standards of practice within the group. Alternative solution: Change the training for and practice of quality assurance.

4. Problem: oversupply of care in some cases. Usual cause: inadequate "utilization controls." Usual solution: Improve utilization controls.

Medical-practice-based cause: To a significant extent, private-practicing physicians create their own demand (Eisenberg; Fuchs and Hahn; Hillman et al.; Leape et al.). They offer a product of which patients have little knowledge (nor do most of them want to acquire it, even if they could). Because of the piecework system of payment, physicians have every incentive to create their own demand. Alternative solution: As above, gradually phase out the piecework system of payment.

5. Problem: the ever-increasing focus on acute-care, high-tech medicine. (This produces the ever-increasing focus on high-tech preservation of fragile biological life at both ends of the age range. This focus gives little consideration to quality-of-life factors or investment in methods which could improve the quality of life without expensive high-tech interventions.) Usual cause: the "technological imperative." Usual solution: There is none; this is a problem we just have to learn to live with (Ginzburg).

Medical-practice-based cause: Rather than being an "imperative" (implying that it somehow has a life of its own), galloping high-tech medicine has been created by a combination of perfectly controllable research, ethical, medical-education-funding, tax, and reimbursement policies. These have had a major influence on medical practice. Alternative solution: Change these policies to stress health promotion, disease and harmful-condition prevention, analysis of cost-benefit and ethical considerations *before* high-tech research and development is undertaken, and rational planning of the distribution and use of high-tech services.

6. Problem: malorganization of the health-care institutional sector. Usual cause: poor planning or the absence of effective free-market influences. Usual solution: Fix the planning system, or let the free market rip.

Medical-practice-base cause: not a major factor in this one, although the overwhelming acute-care bias-emphasis of medical education certainly feeds into it. Alternative solution: re-orient medical education. (But it is surely true that if proactive, not reactive, institutional planning with a separation of institutional capital formation from service reimbursement is not introduced into the system, this problem is insoluble.)

7. Problem: deficiencies in primary care. Usual cause: not enough financial support for primary-care training. Usual solution: Provide some additional funds for primary-care training. Alternatively, spe-

cify a certain number of publicly funded residency training slots for primary care.

Medical-practice-based cause (partial): an undergraduate and graduate medical-education system that emphasizes the specialty approach to medicine not only in its clinical but also its discipline-based basic-science teaching. Alternative solution: Introduce integrated problem-based learning for the basic sciences, and emphasize the practice of medicine, not the diagnosis of organ-based disease, at least in the undergraduate clinical years (AAMC, 1984).

8. Problem: continued presence of "preventable physical pain and mental anguish." Usual cause: lack of reimbursement for preventive services. Usual solution: provision of reimbursement.

Medical-practice-based cause: lack of training in health promotion–disease prevention. If a physician doesn't know how to do it and no interest in it has been generated in the course of his or her training and experience, he or she isn't going to do it, or certainly is not going to do it correctly, whether it's paid for or not. Alternative solution: Change medical education to feature, if not emphasize, health promotion–disease prevention (Jonas, 1978, 1988).

9. Problem: deficiencies in doctor-patient communication. Usual cause: lack of reimbursement for effective communication.

Medical-practice-based cause: similar to that for health promotion/disease prevention—lack of training (and as above). Alternative solution: Change medical education to teach and emphasize the importance of patient-communication skills in all spheres of medical practice (AAMC, 1984).

MAKING EFFECTIVE CHANGE

If this analysis is correct, making change means taking on two of the most powerful institutions in the United States: organized medicine and the possibly even more powerful medical-education establishment (if not more powerful, certainly much less in the public awareness. Its responsibility for the defects in medical practice as well as its great achievements are poorly understood by the general public, most political leaders, and most of the medical-education leadership. This may make it and its inertia even more difficult to change than the AMA.) This is a difficult and daunting task, to say the least.

Neither of the American presidents who had even a notion to take on the medical profession were successful. And they were both strong men. Franklin Roosevelt, like his cousin Teddy in his Bull Moose configuration, wanted national health insurance. But when the AMA threatened to sink Social Security (an interesting moral choice for the representatives of a healing profession) if he did not eliminate NHI from the package, Roosevelt acquiesced. Even in a seemingly favorable postwar climate, Harry Truman went down to defeat on the NHI issue.

But if and when the struggle to change the nature of the practice of medicine does occur, those who lead it are sure to be accused of "doctor bashing." This charge can be dismissed for what it is: a political tactic designed to put the reformers on the defensive and divert attention from the real problems. But beyond that, the kind of analysis engaged in here is not "doctor bashing" of individuals, medical practitioners or medical educators. The problems are with the *systems* of payment and education, not with evil people.

All physicians get caught up in these problems in one way or another. However, the argument should not be seen as a moral one. It is not about right and wrong. It isn't even about "fairness" and "equity." As Dr. Robert M. Sade is fond of pointing out, what one man considers fair another may consider quite unfair. The argument is truly about what works and what doesn't for the health and pocketbook of the people of the United States.

REFERENCES

American Medical Association. *Health Access in America*. Chicago, IL, 1990.

AAMC, Association of American Medical Colleges. *Final Report of the Commission on Medical Education*. New York, 1932.

AAMC. *Physicians for the Twenty-First Century*, report on the panel on the General Education of the Physician (GPEP). Washington, DC, 1984.

Cluff, L. "A Challenge to America's Physicians." *1989 Annual Report*. Princeton, NJ: Robert Wood Johnson Foundation, 1989, pp. 8–11.

Committee on the Costs of Medical Care. *Medical Care for the American People*. Chicago, IL: University of Chicago Press, 1932; reprinted, Washington, DC: U.S. Department of Health Education and Welfare, 1932.

Committee on Labor and Human Resources. *Background Information on S. 1265, The Minimum Health Benefits for All Workers Act of 1988*. Washington, DC: U.S. Senate Committee on Labor and Human Resources, April 29, 1988.

Committee for National Health Insurance. *The Health Security Partnership*. Washington, DC, 1989.

Davis, K., et al. "Paying for Preventive Care: Moving the Debate Forward." *American Journal of Preventive Medicine*, 6(4), suppl., 1990.

Dyckman, Z. *A Study of Physicians' Fees*. Washington, DC: Government Printing Office, 1978.

Eisenberg, J. M. *Doctors' Decisions and the Cost of Medical Care*. Ann Arbor, MI: Health Administration Press Perspectives, 1986.

Fuchs, V. R., & Hahn, J. S. "How Does Canada Do It?" *New England Journal of Medicine, 323*, 884, 1990.

Fuchs, V., & Kramer, M. *Determinants of Expenditures for Physicians' Services in the United States, 1948–68*. Washington, DC: USDHEW Pub. No. (HSM) 73–3013, 1973.

Ginzburg, E. "High-Tech Medicine and Rising Health Care Costs," *Journal of the American Medical Association, 263*, 1820–22, 1990.

Heritage Foundation. *Critical Issues: A National Health System for America*. Washington, DC: Heritage Foundation, 1989.

Hillman, B. J., et al. "Frequency and Costs of Diagnostic Imaging in Office Practice." *New England Journal of Medicine, 323*, 1604, 1990.

Jonas, S. *Medical Mystery: The Training of Doctors in the United States*. New York: W. W. Norton, 1978.

Jonas, S. "Health Promotion in Medical Education." *American Journal of Health Promotion, 3*, 37–42, 51, 1988.

Leape, L. L., et al. "Relation Between Surgeon's Practice Volumes and Geographic Variation in the Rate of Carotid Endarterectomy." *New England Journal of Medicine, 321*, 653, 1989.

MVSR: Monthly Vital Statistics Report. "Advance Report of Final Mortality Statistics, 1988," Vol. 39, No. 7, November 28, 1990.

National Association of Manufacturers. *Meeting the Health Care Crisis*. Washington, DC, 1989.

National Leadership Commission on Health Care. *For the Health of a Nation: A Shared Responsibility*. Ann Arbor, MI: Health Administration Press Perspectives, 1989.

ONCE, Office of National Cost Estimates. "National health expenditures, 1988." *Health Care Financing Review, 11*(4), (Summer 1990), 1–54.

Oil, Chemical and Atomic Workers. *National Health Care: Pass It On!* Lakewood, CO, 1989.

Roemer, M. I. "On Paying the Doctor and the Implications of Different Methods." *Journal of Health and Human Behavior, 3*(4), (Spring 1962).

Rosenthal, E. "Health Problems of Inner City Poor Reach Crisis Point." *The New York Times*, December 24, 1990, p. 1.

Sade, R. M. "A Health-Care Fairy Tale." *Private Practice*, August 1989, pp. 9–17.

Schwartz, E., et al. "Black/White Comparisons of Deaths Preventable by Medical Intervention: United States and the District of Columbia 1980–1986." *International Journal of Epidemiology, 19*, 591, 1990.

USBoC, U.S. Bureau of the Census. *Statistical Abstract of the United States: 1990* (110th edition). Washington, DC: Government Printing Office, 1990.

USPHS, U.S. Public Health Service. *Healthy People 2000: National Health Promotion and Disease Prevention Objectives*, conference ed. Washington, DC., September 1990.

Chapter 8

National Health Insurance

THE WORLD HISTORICAL BACKGROUND

There has been controversy over the issue of national health insurance (NHI) in the United States since the beginning of the twentieth century.* The NHI concept first appeared on the world stage over 100 years ago. Some might be distressed to learn that the content and the form of the arguments for and against it have remained largely fixed. This has been the case regardless of changed circumstances or new information.

The first NHI legislative program was introduced by Otto von Bismarck, the "Iron Chancellor" of Prussia and (after 1871) the unified German state. Shortly after the bourgeois revolution of 1848, he had said: "The social insecurity of the worker is the real cause of their being a peril to the state" (Sigerist, p. 127). In 1881, the German kaiser Wilhelm I, in a speech written by Bismarck, said: "The healing of social evils cannot be sought in the repression of social democratic excesses exclusively but must equally be sought in the positive promotion of the workers' welfare" (Sigerist, p. 129).

Various accident, workers compensation, and sickness schemes, both compulsory and voluntary, had come into existence in the several German states over the previous half century. Building on them, in

---

Health insurance is actually a misnomer. Insurance is the periodic collection of relatively small sums of money from large numbers of people to protect each of them against the financial consequences of a relatively rare event. However, over the course of a lifetime, using health services is not a relatively rare event. Thus "health insurance" is not "insurance" in the conventional sense. Rather it is a system for the collective long-range prepayment of health services. Furthermore, not much "health insurance" money actually pays for health and its promotion. Most of it goes to cover the costs of care during sickness. Nevertheless, as the term is commonly used, so shall it be used in this chapter.

1883 Bismarck succeeded in ushering a Sickness Insurance Act through the German Reichstag (Parliament) (Sigerist, pp. 121–131). Bismarck had wanted a uniform national system, excluding the private, profit-making "sickness societies" (private insurance companies, some profit-making, some not). Understandably, those companies objected to the prospect of being put out of business. In this regard they had much in common with the present U.S. health insurance companies, who protest strongly against any NHI plan that has no role for them.

Bismarck settled for a plan that used the existing network of sickness societies. Nevertheless, it was a national program that paid for medical care and provided cash support during periods of sickness and accidental injury for certain categories of workers. Two-thirds of the premiums were paid by the employees, one-third by the employers. Thus the first national health insurance scheme was created not by a progressive democratic or socialist government but a conservative monarchy.

By the 1920s, most European industrialized countries and Japan had some kind of national health insurance system. It usually began as a partial and/or voluntary system, generally progressing to a comprehensive and compulsory one (Douglas-Wilson & McLachlan, pp. 1–123, 211–230; Fry & Farndale; Glaser; Roemer). After World War II, the English-speaking British Commonwealth countries gradually followed suit (Fry & Farndale; Lynch & Raphael; Roemer). The United States is the only industrialized country in the world other than South Africa without some sort of NHI system (see Chapter 9).

THE HISTORY OF NHI IN THE UNITED STATES

The first campaign for a national health insurance program in the United States was undertaken by the American Association for Labor Legislation (AALL), a middle-class, liberal, reform-minded group founded in 1906 (Anderson, Pt. 2; Burrow, 1963; 1977, pp. 138–153). Proposals for a broad social insurance plan were part of Teddy Roosevelt's Bull Moose (third) party platform in 1912 (Burrow, 1963, p. 135). In 1916, the AALL proposed a standard bill for compulsory medical care and sickness-benefits insurance, suggesting that the states adopt the program independently. It would have covered persons earning below a certain income level and used existing insurance carriers. Employers, employees, and the states would have shared the costs (Anderson, pp. 62–65; Burrow, 1963, p. 136).

At first, support was widespread, extending to the American Medical Association and even the National Association of Manufacturers (Burrow, 1963, pp. 138–145). Beginning in 1917, however, when the United States entry into World War I was deflating the reform movement generally, opposition began to surface from several quarters. Among the opponents were the American Federation of Labor and the commercial insurance industry (Anderson, p. 67; Burrow, 1977, pp. 148–153).

Within the AMA, a battle ensued (Anderson; Burrow, 1963, pp. 146–151). As part of a general takeover of power by the practitioner wing from the academic wing, the conservative faction won out (Harris, p. 30).* In 1920, the AMA House of Delegates passed the following resolution (Burrow, 1963, p. 150):

> Resolved, that the American Medical Association declares its opposition to the institution of any plan embodying the system of compulsory contributory insurance against illness, or any other plan of compulsory insurance which provides for medical service to be rendered contributors or their dependents, provided, controlled, or regulated by any state or the Federal government.

That remained the AMA position until the late 1960s (Harris). Even in the mid-1970s, by which time the AMA had adopted an NHI proposal of its own that ran counter to the bulk of the 1920 resolution, the "noncompulsory" principle was retained (Committee on Ways and Means). By 1990, the AMA had also dropped the noncompulsory principle (AMA, 1990).

Serious consideration was next given to national health insurance during the development of the Social Security Act of 1935. This consideration was stimulated in part by the final report of the Committee on the Costs of Medical Care (1932; see also Anderson; Stevens, pp. 183–187). In 1934, President Franklin Roosevelt created the Committee on Economic Security to consider the question of social insurance.

NHI did not last long on the agenda. The principal opposition came from the American Medical Association (Burrow, 1963, p. 193). The committee's executive director, Edwin E. Witte, wrote (Anderson, p. 108):

---

*Both Burrow's book and the Harris articles contain detailed histories and analyses of the AMA's involvement in legislative battles over NHI. The 1963 Burrow book details them through the 1950s. The Harris articles cover the Medicare struggles. An excellent overall historical perspective is provided by Falk (1977).

When in 1934 the Committee on Economic Security announced that it was studying health insurance, it was at once subjected to misrepresentation and vilification. In the original social security bill there was one line to the effect that the Social Security Board should study the problem and make a report thereon to Congress. That little line was responsible for so many telegrams to the members of Congress that the entire social security program seemed endangered until the Ways and Means Committee unanimously struck it out of the bill.

The president wanted the basic Social Security Act, one of the cornerstones of the New Deal. It was passed with no reference to NHI.*

Senator Robert F. Wagner, Sr. of New York initiated the next major legislative foray. His landmark Wagner Act of 1938 had established the right to collective bargaining for all nonpublic employees in the United States. In 1939, he introduced a bill (Sigerist, pp. 189–190) "to provide for the general welfare by enabling the several states to make more adequate provision for public health, prevention and control of disease, maternal and child health services, construction, and maintenance of needed hospitals and health centers, care of the sick, disability insurance, and training of personnel."

The bill, S. 1620, proposed to subsidize state public health programs (this later became federal policy through a series of separate acts); the construction of hospitals (enacted in 1946 as the Hill-Burton Act); and state programs for medical care for the poor (eventually enacted in part in 1960 as the "Kerr/Mills" Medical Assistance for the Aged, then expanded as Medicaid in 1965). The bill also offered cash sickness benefits (a standard feature of the European-Japanese approach to NHI that has never made headway in the United States). Also there was to be a program of federal subsidies to those states enacting comprehensive health insurance programs (Harris, pp. 31–32; Sigerist, pp. 190–191). The bill died in committee after being vigorously attacked by the AMA (Harris, pp. 38–40).

Senator Wagner tried again in 1943, this time in concert with Senator Murray and Representative Dingell. Their S. 1161 "advocated a national (i.e., Federal) compulsory system of health insurance, financed from payroll taxes and providing comprehensive health and medical benefits through entitlement to specified medical service benefits" (Stevens, p. 272). This was the first major legislative proposal for a federal rather than a state system.

---

*The details of all major NHI proposals made between 1935 and 1957 have been summarized in A. W. Brewster, *Health Insurance and Related Proposals for Financing Personal Health Services* (Washington, DC: Government Printing Office, 1958).

Once again, the AMA responded with vigor (Harris, pp. 40–42). The bill never got very far, although it was reintroduced in several successive congresses (Anderson, pp. 112–113). In 1947, Senator Robert Taft, Sr., first introduced a Medicaidlike proposal for federal subsidies to the states to pay for medical care for the poor (Stevens, p. 273). Though sponsored by a conservative Republican, it also got nowhere.

In 1949 Harry Truman, reelected president with Democratic majorities in both houses of Congress, decided to make enactment of NHI a major goal of his administration. He proposed a national compulsory system, to be paid for by a combination of Social Security and general taxation. It was to be based upon the following principles, which he had originally enunciated in 1945 (Truman, 1958, pp. 629–630):

> Everyone should have ready access to all necessary medical, hospital, and related services. . . . A system of required prepayment would not only spread the costs of medical care, it would also prevent much serious disease. . . . Such a system of prepayment should cover medical, hospital, nursing, and laboratory services. It should cover dental care [as far as] resources of the system permit. . . . The nation-wide system must be highly decentralized in administration. . . . Subject to national standards, methods and rates of paying doctors and hospitals should be adjusted locally. . . . People should remain free to choose their own physicians and hospitals. . . . Likewise physicians should remain free to accept or reject patients. . . . Our voluntary hospitals and our city, county, and state general hospitals, in the same way, must be free to participate in the system to whatever extent they wish. . . . What I am recommending is not socialized medicine. Socialized medicine means that all doctors work as employees of government. . . . No such system is proposed.

Does this statement not have a highly contemporary ring to it?

The AMA mounted a furious attack on the plan, based primarily on the thesis that it was indeed "socialized medicine" (Harris, pp. 40–62). The AMA used a major public relations firm and a war chest of over $2 million, a substantial sum in those days, and with allies from the drug and insurance industries (Stevens, pp. 273–274), it was once again successful. With the election of a Republican government in 1952, the AMA was able to breathe easily (Burrow, 1963, pp. 361, 385).

In the post–World War II climate of domestic and foreign anti-communism (Freeland), it was difficult for Truman to win support at home for a program consistently attacked as "communist" or at least "socialist," but in any case "red" (Harris, p. 50). Thus, in 1951, on the recommendation of Oscar Ewing, then federal security administrator, the Truman administration withdrew its support for NHI and began the campaign that led to the passage of Medicare, limited health insurance for the aged, in 1965 (Harris, pp. 58–60; Stevens, p. 274).

MEDICARE AND MEDICAID

The campaign for Medicare was long and arduous (Harris; Stevens, pp. 432–443). It met with success in 1965 (Committee on Finance, 1970). Both Medicare and its afterthought companion Medicaid (Friedman) had historical antecedents. In most countries where the central government has undertaken NHI, it began by taking care of only part of the population, usually low-income persons (as in Medicaid). In the United States, the earliest AALL proposals contained the concept of beginning with partial coverage. However, the AALL programs were aimed at the working poor, whereas Medicaid covers primarily the nonworking poor. Medicaidlike proposals had appeared in Senator Wagner's prewar bill and Senator Taft's postwar bills. Determination of an eligible population by age was, however, a new twist, going back only to 1950.

NATIONAL HEALTH INSURANCE IN THE 1960s AND 1970s

Beginning in the late 1960s, many new legislative proposals for NHI were made (Burns; Eilers; Falk, 1977; New York Academy of Medicine). In the 1970s, they were summarized by the Ways and Means Committee of the House of Representatives (e.g., Committee on Ways and Means, 1974), the Senate Finance Committee (Committee on Finance, 1979), and Davis (1975). As noted above, in the wide-ranging debate on NHI, the basic arguments of the several sides had changed little over time (Boas; Falk, 1973; McKittrick; H. Schwartz).

As of 1975, a time when the passage of some sort of NHI seemed imminent to many observers, there were four major proposals before Congress. The constituencies represented were organized labor, the American Hospital Association, the Health Insurance Association of America, and (by this time) the AMA. Since all the major actors were on stage, it was believed that surely one of these proposals or some compromise would find its way through Congress.

One predicts the passage of National Health Insurance in the United States at one's peril, however. For example, in 1974, an observer wrote (Jonas, 1974): "The United States of America is the only major country in the developed, capitalist world without some form of national health insurance programme. The struggle for national health insurance in the U.S., a long and bitter one, has been well described. It now appears as if there will be some form of national health insurance legislation in the U.S. *before the Presidential elections of 1976* [emphasis added]." There wasn't.

In the 1976 presidential campaign, candidate Jimmy Carter said in his only speech on health policy (*Nation's Health*, 1976, p. 7):

> We must have a comprehensive program of national health insurance. . . . The coverage must be universal and mandatory. We must lower the present barriers, in insurance coverage and otherwise, to preventive and primary care and thus reduce the need for hospitalization. We must have strong cost and quality controls, and . . . rates . . . should be set in advance. . . . We must phase in the program as rapidly as revenues permit, helping first those who need help, and achieving a comprehensive program well defined in the end.

His administration never submitted comprehensive NHI legislation to Congress.

NATIONAL HEALTH INSURANCE PROPOSALS IN THE 1980s

In 1979 the Congressional Research Service of the Library of Congress (Cavalier) stated that the major policy issues to be addressed in designing an NHI program were:

1. The rising costs of health care.
2. The gaps in present health insurance coverage in services and populations.
3. Geographic maldistribution of personnel and facilities.
4. Access to service by ability to pay, social class, age group, and geography.
5. The impact, or lack thereof, of NHI on the population's health status.

A familiar-sounding problem list. No one attended to it.

In 1980 the same major players were still on the field (Committee on Finance, 1979; Kimble; pp. 448–453 of the 2nd ed. of *Health Care*

Delivery in the United States). But with the election of Ronald Reagan in 1980, the whole movement ran out of gas.

A measure of the enormous loss of energy suffered by the pro-NHI forces in the 1980s can be found in the contents of the "reform package" offered in 1985 by Senator Kennedy (with Representative Fortney "Pete" Stark, House Ways and Means Committee, Health Subcommittee Chair). They proposed (*Washington Report on Medicine & Health*, 1985):

1. To reduce the number of persons uninsured for health-care costs by requiring employers to make health insurance available to former employees at group rates.
2. To reduce or eliminate "patient dumping" by hospitals.
3. To restrain increases in Medicare Part A premium costs.
4. To hold down Medicare payments to hospitals.

This was a far cry from the sweeping changes proposed by Kennedy in several bills he offered in the 1970s.

NHI BY CONTRACT, OR THE PERSONAL HEALTH CARE SYSTEM

In the early 1980s a proposal designed to deal with the problem list set out by the Congressional Research Service and many others was published (Jonas, 1981, 1984). First designated NHI by Contract, more recently it has been called the Personal Health Care System (PHCS). By 1991, it had yet to be put into legislative language.

A classical approach to the achievement of stated goals and objectives is the contract mechanism. The buyer and seller of a product agree on product or service specifications and costs in the contract. The contract usually contains means of enforcement of its terms. A small-scale, partial prototype of such an approach to the financing, planning, and evaluation of health services existed in New York City during the 1970s (Jonas, 1977), known colloquially as ghetto medicine.

Under NHI by Contract, PHCS, government would raise the funds necessary to pay for health services. It would then negotiate a series of contracts with providers, who would agree to offer a set of services to the population for a given sum. Most existing providers, institutional or individual, would be eligible to become either primary contractors or subcontractors. In this, NHI by Contract has much in common with the health-care-corporation concept of the mid-1970s, an American Hospital Association plan.

The composition of the service packages would be determined by health-planning mechanisms. There would be free competition among the providers for the contracts, with bidders offering to provide the specified services at varying prices. Primary contractors would be paid on a global-budget basis. Much as group-practice and independent health maintenance organizations do now, all contractors would then market their services to consumers.

All persons would be covered by a benefit package that would be determined nationally. Consumers would have free choice of contractor, but once having made their choice, as in present dual-choice situations, patients would have to stay with the selected provider for a minimium period. Advisory boards consisting of patients served by each contractor would be formed. The consumer role would focus on the evaluation of outcomes, that is, the extent to which contractors met their contract specifications. The boards would be party to contract negotiation and enforcement. There would be graded financial penalties for failure to meet contract specifications and rewards for excellent performance. Private ownership of the health-services sector, including private medical practice, would be maintained. But the people, through the government and the advisory boards, would have a strong voice in deciding how their money would be spent.

Government would have three principal roles: raiser of funds, negotiator of contracts, and enforcer of contracts (in concert with the advisory boards). Government responsibilities would be distributed among national, state, and local jurisdictions. The system would be supported by a combination of employer-employee contributions and general tax revenues. Technology assessment, carried out at the federal level, would provide important data for health planning and priority setting. Insurance companies could be used as fiscal intermediaries.

NHI by Contract provides the opportunity to deal directly with most of the principal problems presently facing the U.S. health-care system, including cost control; quality improvement; implementing a comprehensive health-promotion and disease-prevention program; introducing rationality into the planning, development, and use of personnel and physical resources; and achieving equity of access. It enables the direct focusing of effort and payment. A fair degree of fine-tuning can be accomplished.

PHCS leaves behind the present reliance on regulation and prayer to achieve program goals and objectives. It does not begin with benefit packages and decisions on copayment, like so many other approaches to NHI. It starts with the establishment of planning principles. It assumes that benefit packages will be developed and decisions on copayment made after needs are assessed, goals and objectives set, and the amount of available funds determined. Then the contract specifications will be written, balancing needs, priorities, and available funds.

PHCS would provide an integral link between the planning and financing of health services. As Rashi Fein, chair of the Institute of Medicine's Committee on Health Planning Goals and Standards, noted in his preface to the committee's report, this is essential to problem solving (IOM, vol. 1, p. iii): "The committee believes that the forces at work in the American health care system, including the various reimbursement mechanisms, cannot be countered by a health planning effort that is divorced, among other limiting factors, from the flow of funds."

Using epidemiological methods in health-services planning, PHCS would carry out ongoing needs assessments, set priorities based on them, and within the limits of available resources, make continual program adjustments to meet identified needs. The approach would allow for the direct application of planning information to health services. Thus the focus on meeting identified needs could always be maintained without direct government services.

The assumption is made that the numerous individual health-care providers are incapable of rational planning on their own (the history of "voluntarism" in health planning has shown that this is true); thus, government action in this area is necessary. It also is assumed (as it is in most other NHI proposals) that government will play an increasingly important role in the financing of health services, whether through taxation or the imposition and collection of uniform employer-employee contributions to pay for the cost of health services.

PHCS would:

1. Maintain the present pattern of ownership of health facilities.
2. Probably but not necessarily change the employment patterns of personnel presently engaged in fee-for-service practice.
3. Provide for the continued existence of the insurance companies in reduced size.
4. Place government at arms's length from the direct operation of health services.
5. Provide a significant role for consumers in health services evaluation, by outcomes.

The system would probably be quite cumbersome, especially for the first few years. Negotiations would be extremely complex. Long lead times, to which few Americans are accustomed, would be required for their conclusion. The providers would be called upon to make functional and psychological changes, although not of the same magnitude as would be required under a national health service. Behavioral change would also be required among patients, although experience with HMOs indicates that patient behavioral change would come more easily than provider behavioral change. From the perspective of most patients, the PHCS would look a great deal like a vastly expanded HMO system. There would be a large pool of staff in the health insurance industry that would have to be laid off or reassigned as individual claims processing became a thing of the past. However, there would be many new positions in negotiating bodies at many levels and in inspectorates.

NATIONAL HEALTH INSURANCE IN THE 1990s

For a variety of reasons, (primarily continually escalating costs, a growing pool of uninsured persons, and declining health for certain portions of the population; see also the problem lists in Chapters 1 and 7), NHI is once again on the national agenda. Once again there are a series of proposals on the table from such disparate groups as Senator Kennedy's Committee on Labor and Human Resources (1988), the National Association of Manufacturers (1989), the Heritage Foundation (1989), the National Leadership Commission on Health Care (cochaired by former presidents Nixon, Ford, and Carter), the Oil, Chemical and Atomic Workers (1989), the Committee for National Health Insurance (affiliated with the AFL-CIO) (1989), the American Medical Association (AMA), the American Public Health Association (*The Nation's Health*), the U.S. Bipartisan Commission on Comprehensive Health Care of the U.S. Congress (known as the Pepper Commission) (1990), and the Physicians for a National Health Program (Himmelstein & Woolhandler).

As noted in Chapter 7, the proposals are primarily formalistic rather than substantive; they deal with the conditions of medical practice, not with medical practice itself. Among many reformers there seems almost to be a fear of taking on the medical profession. Well-known promoters of change look almost anywhere else for the cause of the problems (see for example Ehrenreich, 1990, who labeled the insurance industry the villain of the piece, as if it practiced and spent health-care dollars instead of just transferring them from patient-payor to provider).

NHI in Canada

What eventually became a national health insurance program for Canada began in one province, Saskatchewan, in 1947.* Nationwide coverage for hospital care was introduced in 1957, followed by coverage for physicians' services in 1971. The Canadian experience with NHI has generated much interest in the United States, both pro and con (Evans, et al.; Fuchs & Hahn; Goodman; *Hospitals;* Igelhart, 1986, 1990; Linton; Woolhandler & Himmelstein). The present Canadian system has been in place for about 20 years. It is founded on four principles:

1. Universal coverage for all Canadians, with low or no copayments and reasonable access to care.
2. The benefits for each covered person are portable from province to province.
3. All medically necessary services are covered.
4. Administration is by not-for-profit public agencies.

In practice, this means that all acute-care and certain long-term services are covered. The provincial governments run the program and pay for about 65 percent of all hospital and medical care. Private insurance is limited to noncovered services (e.g., some dental and some long-term care). The program is funded is primarily from progressive taxation at both the federal and provincial levels. Several provinces do charge premiums, either at a flat rate or in proportion to wages (up to a maximum).

Most hospitals are private, not-for-profit. Most doctors are in private practice. The plans pay the hospitals with a lump-sum budget to cover all operating expenses (the payments are made every few weeks). Capital funds come from the insurance fund but are allocated to hospitals separately from their expense budgets (in that way, the plan keeps control of hospital capital expenditure, an essential element of any effective cost-containment program). Patients are billed only for items deemed "luxury," such as elective private rooms.

Physicians are paid on a fee-for-service basis, according to a fee

---

*This section is based in part on a personal communication from Dr. Milton Roemer, February 5, 1991.

schedule negotiated between the provinces and the medical societies. They can bill only for their personal services, not the capital costs of machinery in their private offices or the work of other health professionals. Physicians cannot "balance-bill" (charge a patient extra for any service covered by the plan). In American terminology, Canadian physicians must "accept assignment" (agree to be paid by the plan, not the patient). Patients have freedom of choice of provider.

Access to care has improved dramatically over the years. Most measures of health are as good or better than those in the United States. Cost increases have been relatively modest. In the 1960s, the percentage of GNP spent for health care was about the same in Canada and the United States. By 1989, it was over 30 percent higher in the latter (see Chapter 5). Medicine has remained a desirable profession in Canada. In 1987, the ratio of applicants to available medical-school spaces was 4.7 in Canada, compared with 1.8 in the U.S.

Canadian physician incomes have remained about where they were before NHI, around 4.8 times the average industrial wage. That level is about the same as (reported) physician income here. Income differentials between primary-care and specialist physicians are rather low (unlike the situation in the United States). There is considerably less bureaucratic interference in clinical practice in Canada, and billing is considerably simpler. Out of about 50,000 physicians in Canada, in 1985 fewer than 400 chose to emigrate to the United States.

There are problems. There has been some rationing (some call it prudent use) of certain high-tech services. There has been some overservicing by physicians (responded to by the institution of a total-income pool and physician income caps). There is some geographic maldistribution of physicians, but it has been reduced. (Responses to that problem have been the two tried and true methods of national health care systems: bonuses for going to underserved areas and banning from overserved areas.) Long-term care is uneven among the provinces, but generally it has been improved. Prevention still does not receive adequate attention, although its status is better too. The nurse-population ratio is the highest in the world. Thus there is little use of allied health professionals.

Cost containment has been achieved by:

1. Eliminating the payment middlemen or reducing their number to one.
2. Eliminating the private insurance companies from any piece of the action other than supplementary insurance.

3. Having a single source of payment (the "monopsony payor"), which can set limits on total payments while making some choices about what the payments are made for.
4. Separating out hospital capital formation. (Hospital operating policies therefore do not have to be tailored to create capital funds or pay off loans, for example by encouraging reimbursable procedure-based interventions. Capital investment can then be planned on the basis of unmet-need analysis.)
5. A reimbursement system for hospitals, global budgeting, which rewards neither over- nor underutilization and encourages "prudent" management, although extraordinary payments are in extraordinary circumstances.
6. Controlling payments to physicians through use of a fee schedule and mandatory assignment.

The key features of the Canadian system that differ from that of the United States are:

1. Global budgeting for hospitals.
2. A combination of fee-for-service private practice with mandatory assignment, no balance billing, and possible income caps.
3. Elimination for the insurance companies.
4. Prospective, external, community-needs-based planning for capital-investment decisions and separation of capital expenditure from operational expenditures.

The major lessons to learn from the Canadian experience are not the details of the system (what level of government runs it, who administers it, exactly what the benefits are, exactly what the sources of revenue are, exactly how services are billed, and so forth). They are, first, that government has a major role to play in the operation of any smoothly functioning health-care delivery system, although it certainly does not have to own and run the system. Both ownership and operating responsibility can remain in private hands as long as everyone is on the same page and government assembles the resources and sets the limits (rather than having the "free market" set them).

Second, we should learn that if changes are to have any utility, we must first determine and analyze the true causes of the problems we are setting out to solve. We must aim our solutions at those causes, as the Canadians have done. U.S. reformers only weaken their position by extolling the virtues of the Canadian system to the extent that they must spend most of their time defending that system. It appears to be more useful to undertake a causal analysis of the problems in the U.S. system, perhaps as has been done in Chapter 7, and develop U.S. solutions to them, using the Canadian experience as a guide.

LOOKING AHEAD

It is popular in some circles to say that NHI is too expensive, that the nation cannot afford it. According to proponents of the comprehensive plans, the truth is just the opposite. They say that with the skyrocketing costs, questionable quality, increases in preventable death in certain segments of the population (*MVSR;* Rosenthal; E. Schwartz et al.), and massive misallocation of resources that occur under the present voluntary "free" system, the nation cannot afford *not* to have it. However, it must be recognized that any NHI plan that does not tackle the *causes* of the problems head-on, any plan that just pays in a different way for the system we now have, will in the long run probably make things worse. We must not pay differently for things: We must pay for different things.

Making change in the U.S. health-care system is difficult, as history has taught us again and again. The provider groups are powerful, the two most powerful the physicians and the hospitals. In the past, major changes in the system have taken place when physicians and/ or hospitals wanted or needed those changes. Examples include the reinstitution of medical licensing laws and the reduction in the number of medical schools in the late nineteenth and early twentieth centuries, and the development of voluntary hospital insurance during the Great Depression. NHI will probably come when one or both of those groups want it or need it.

The private hospitals will want it when an increasing number of them go bankrupt in the face of uncontrolled cost increases and declining occupancy rates, as happened in Great Britain just before the institution of its National Health Service in 1948. The physicians will want it when their numbers are so large that they will no longer be able to sell all the product they can collectively produce as they can now. If a majority were still private entrepreneurs at that time, the competition would be chaotic (Consumer Commission). The shelter of a secure if somewhat smaller income would be sought in salaried service.

Proposals for solutions abound. None of them are perfect in anyone's eyes; however, some of them have more potential for solving the major problems than others. Those with the most potential have one key characteristic in common: proactive, not reactive, planning, linked to financing. As Blum has asked, however, "Can there be meaningful health planning [in the United States] when so little else is planned?"

The resistance to planning in the health-care industry is particularly strong. For example, in the fall of 1985, then Senator Dan Quayle (R, Ind.) proposed the creation of a national advisory council to make recommendations for minimum percentages of primary-care-specialty residency positions in the several classes of teaching hospitals. This system would have been entirely voluntary (when a mandatory health personnel supply, distribution, and allocation system is needed). The united reaction from the American Medical Association, the American Hospital Association, and the Association of American Medical Colleges was a resounding and vehement no (Association of American Medical Colleges, 1985). The present personnel situation is chaotic and wasteful. It has been created by 50 years of individually isolated unplanned action. But the three leading health-care organizations rejected even an advisory system dealing with only one piece of the pie.

Finally, if there is no planning, no system, no national program, what will happen? Some predict major catastrophe and crisis. But in spite of predictions of impending doom going back 20 years and more (see Chapter 1), no national catastrophe has occurred (although millions of individuals have suffered). The system just keeps barreling along, getting ever more expensive and showing major defects in the quality and the quantity of service provided. Will there be a crisis? Will there be a catastrophe? Or will we just continue to experience more of the same? The outcome of this drama is one that no one can predict.

REFERENCES

AMA, American Medical Association. *Health Access America*. Chicago, March 1990.

Anderson, O. W. *The Uneasy Equilibrium: Private and Public Financing of Health Services in the United States, 1875–1965*. New Haven, CT: College and University Press, 1968.

Association of American Medical Colleges. "AMA/AHA/AAMC Object to Bill on Medical Education." *Weekly Report*, September 26, 1985, p. 2.

Blum, H. L. "*Health Planning: Lessons for the Future*, by Bonnie Lefkowitz" (book review). *Inquiry*, 20, 390, 1983.

Boas, F. P. *Why Do We Need National Health Insurance?* Society for Ethical Culture, 1945. Reprinted in Committee on Medical Care Teaching of the Association of Teachers of Preventive Medicine, *Readings in Medical Care.* Chapel Hill: University of North Carolina Press, 1958.

Burns, E. M. "Health Insurance: Not If, or When, But What Kind?" *American Journal of Public Health, 61,* 2164, 1971.

Burrow, J. G. *AMA: Voice of American Medicine.* Baltimore: Johns Hopkins University Press, 1963.

Burrow, J. G. *Organized Medicine in the Progressive Era.* Baltimore: Johns Hopkins University Press, 1977.

Cavalier, K. *National Health Insurance.* Washington DC: Congressional Research Service, Library of Congress, 1979.

Committee on the Costs of Medical Care. *Medical Care for the American People.* Chicago: University of Chicago Press, 1932; reprinted Washington, DC: USDHEW, 1970.

Committee on Finance, United States Senate. *Medicare and Medicaid: Problems, Issues and Alternatives.* Washington, DC: Government Printing Office, 1970.

Committee on Finance, United States Senate. *Comparison of Major Features of Health Insurance Proposals.* Washington, DC: Government Printing Office, 1979.

Committee on Labor and Human Resources. *Background Information on S. 1265, The Minimum Health Benefits for All Workers Act of 1988.* Washington, DC: US Senate Committee on Labor and Human Resources, April 29, 1988.

Committee for National Health Insurance. *The Health Security Partnership,* Washington, DC: 1989.

Committee on Ways and Means, House of Representatives. *National Health Insurance Resource Book.* Washington, DC: Government Printing Office, 1974.

Consumer Commission on the Accreditation of Health Services. "National Health Service V: Building a Medical Staff." *Consumer Health Perspectives, 5*(3), 1, 1978.

Davis, K. *National Health Insurance: Benefits, Costs, and Consequences.* Washington, DC: Brookings Institution, 1975.

Douglas-Wilson, I., & McLachlan, G. *Health Service Prospects: An International Survey.* Boston: Little, Brown, 1973.

Eilers, R. D. "National Health Insurance: What Kind and How Much? Parts 1 and 2." *New England Journal of Medicine, 284,* 881, 945, 1971.

Ehrenreich, B. "Our Health-Care Disgrace." *Time,* December 10, 1990, p. 112.

Evans, R. G., et al. "Controlling Health Expenditures—The Canadian Reality," *New England Journal of Medicine, 320,* 571, 1989.

Falk, I. S. "Medical Care in the USA, 1932–1972. Problems, Proposals and Programs from the Committee on the Costs of Medical Care to the Committee for National Health Insurance." *Health and Society, 51,* 1, 1973.

Falk, I. S. "Proposals of Nation Health Insurance in the USA: Origins and Evolution, and Some Perceptions for the Future." *Health and Society*, Spring 1977, p. 161.

Freeland, R. M. *The Truman Doctrine and the Origins of McCarthyism*. New York: Knopf, 1975.

Friedman, E. "Medicaid." Part 1, *Hospitals, 51*, August 16, 1977, p. 51, (a); Part 2, *Hospitals, 51*, September 1, 1977, p. 59, (b); Part 3, *Hospitals, 51*, September 16, 1977, p. 73 (c); Part 4, *Hospitals, 51*, October 1, 1977, p. 61, (d); Part 5, *Hospitals, 51*, November 1, 1977, p. 77, (e).

Fry, J., & Farndale, W. A. J., eds. *International Medical Care*. Oxford, England: MTP, 1972.

Fuchs, V. R., & Hahn, J. S. "How Does Canada Do It?" *New England Journal of Medicine, 323*, 884, 1990.

Glaser, W. A. *Health Insurance Bargaining*. New York: Gardner Press, 1978.

Goodman, W. E. "Canada's Health-Care System: You Get What You Pay For." *Private Practice*, October 1989, p. 11.

Harris, R. "Annals of Legislation: Medicare." *The New Yorker*, July 2, July 9, July 16, July 23, 1966.

Heritage Foundation. *Critical Issues: A National Health System for America*, Washington, DC: Heritage Foundation, 1989.

Himmelstein, D. U., & Woolhandler, S. "A National Health Program for the United States." *New England Journal of Medicine, 320*, 102, 1989 [a].

Hospitals. "The Delivery Challenges Posed by Canada: A Bilateral View," November 5, 1990, p. 58.

Igelhart, J. "Canada's Health Care System" (Parts 1, 2, 3). *New England Journal of Medicine, 315*, 202, 778, 1623, 1986.

Igelhart, J. "Canada's Health Care System Faces Its Problems." *New England Journal of Medicine, 322*, 562, 1990.

IOM, Institute of Medicine, Committee on Health Planning Goals and Standards. *Health Planning in the United States: Selected Policy Issues*. 2 Vols. Washington, DC: National Academy Press, 1981.

Jonas, S. "Issues in National Health Insurance in the United States of America." *The Lancet*, July 20, 1974, p. 143.

Jonas, S. *Quality-Control of Ambulatory Care*. New York: Springer Publishing Co., 1977.

Jonas, S. "Planning for National Health Insurance by Objective: The Contract Mechanism." In R. Straetz, ed., *Critical Perspectives and Issues in Health Policy*. Lexington, MA: Lexington Books, 1981.

Jonas, S. "The Personal Health Care System." *New York State Journal of Medicine, 84*, 187, 1984.

Kimble, C. "Special Report: Comparing the Carter and Kennedy National Health Insurance Bills." *Washington Report on Medicine and Health*, November 1979.

Linton, A. L. "The Canadian Health Care System: A Canadian Physician's Perspective." *New England Journal of Medicine, 322*, 197, 1990.

Lynch, M. J., & Raphael, S. S. *Medicine and the State*. Springfield, IL: Charles C. Thomas, 1963.

McKittrick, L. S. "Medical Care for the American People: Is Compulsory Health Insurance the Solution?" *New England Journal of Medicine, 240,* 998, 1949. Reprinted in Committee on Medical Care Teaching of the Association of Teachers of Preventive Medicine. *Readings in Medical Care.* Chapel Hill: University of North Carolina Press, 1958.

MVSR, Monthly Vital Statistics Report. "Advance Report of Final Mortality Statistics, 1988," *39* (7), Suppl., November 28, 1990.

National Association of Manufacturers. *Meeting the Health Care Crisis.* Washington, DC, 1989.

National Leadership Commission on Health Care. *For the Health of a Nation: A Shared Responsibility.* Ann Arbor, MI: Health Administration Press Perspectives, 1989.

The Nation's Health. "Carter Addresses Annual Meeting." November, 1976, p. 1.

The Nation's Health. "Insurance Plan Stresses Reform, Prevention," March, 1990, p. 1.

New York Academy of Medicine. "Toward a National Health Program." *Bulletin of New York Academy of Medicine, 48,* January 1972.

Oil, Chemical and Atomic Workers. *National Health Care: Pass It On!* Lakewood, CO, 1989.

Roemer, M. I. "I. S. Falk, the Committee on the Costs of Medical Care, and the Drive for National Health Insurance." *American Journal of Public Health, 75,* 841, 1985.

Rosenthal, E. "Health Problems of the Inner City Poor Reach Crisis Point." *The New York Times,* December 24, 1990, p. 1.

Schwartz, E., et al. "Black/White Comparisons of Deaths Preventable by Medical Intervention: United States and the District of Columbia 1980–86." *International Journal of Epidemiology, 19,* 591, 1990.

Schwartz, H. *The Case for American Medicine: A Realistic Look at Our Health Care System.* New York: David McKay, 1972.

Sigerist, H. E. *On the Sociology of Medicine,* ed. M. I. Roemer. New York: MD Publications, 1960.

Stevens, R. *American Medicine and the Public Interest.* New Haven, CT: Yale University Press, 1971.

Truman, H. S. *Message from the President of the United States.* 79th Congress, 1st Session. Washington, DC: Government Printing Office, 1945. Reprinted in Committee on Medical Care Teaching. *Readings in Medical Care.* Chapel Hill: University of North·Carolina Press, 1958.

U.S. Bipartisan Commission on Comprehensive Health Care. *A Call for Action.* Washington, DC: Government Printing Office, September 1990.

Washington Report on Medicine and Health. "Stark, Kennedy to Propose Health Reforms," June 17, 1985.

Woolhandler, S., & Himmelstein, D. U. "Resolving the Cost/Access Conflict." *Journal of General Internal Medicine, 4,* 54, 1989.

Chapter **9**

National Health Systems throughout the World

Milton I. Roemer

Every country has a national health system that reflects its history, economic development, and dominant political ideology. Because of these diverse circumstances, there are several types of health systems, the highlights of which this chapter will examine in industrialized and developing countries. The type of health system depends on the characteristics of the system's component parts.

COMPOSITION OF HEALTH SYSTEMS

Any national health system in a country at any stage of economic development may be analyzed according to five principal component parts: (1) resources, (2) organization, (3) management, (4) economic support, and (5) delivery of services. The resources of a health system consist of human resources (personnel), facilities (hospitals, health centers, etc.), commodities (drugs, equipment, supplies, etc.), and knowledge. Each of these may be produced or acquired in different ways and to various extents. Health programs may be organized under diverse sponsorships: one principal authority of government (at several levels), other governmental agencies with health functions, voluntary health agencies, enterprises, and a private health-care market. The proportions among these five major forms of organization vary greatly in different countries.

The management of health systems entails several processes: health planning, administration (supervision, consultation, co-ordination, etc.), regulation, and legislation. The methods of carrying out each managerial process tend to vary mainly with a country's dominant political ideology. The economic support of the various parts of a health system usually depends on one of more financial mechanisms. These may be governmental tax revenues (at different levels), social insurance (statutory), voluntary insurance, charity, and personal households. In economically less developed countries, for-eign aid may play a role. The relative proportions among these different forms of support influence many features of a health system.

Finally, these four component parts of a health system lead to the crucial fifth part: the delivery of health services, which may be analyzed according to three main subdivisions: primary health care (preventive and curative), secondary care, and tertiary care. In most health systems, furthermore, there are special modes of delivery of health services to certain populations and for certain disorders.

The combined characteristics of these five component parts permit the designation of each national health system according to certain *types*. While history, economic level, and political ideology determine these types, their attributes may be classified according to the degree of *market intervention by government*. The organization of every health system includes a private health care market. The proportions and characteristics of this market depend on the extent of intervention in the market process—supply, demand, competition, and price—by government. This may be measured, as we shall see, in different ways appropriate to each component.

By such analysis, the national health systems in the world's ap-proximately 165 sovereign countries may be scaled into four main types. Going from the least market intervention to the most, these health-system types are (1) entrepreneurial, (2) welfare-oriented, (3) comprehensive, and (4) socialist. This scaling may be applied, fur-thermore, to countries at high, middle, and low levels of economic development. In this chapter, we examine health systems in illustra-tive industrialized countries and in selected developing countries of both middle and low economic levels. Health systems change over time, and this article describes the situation in the late 1980s.

ENTREPRENEURIAL HEALTH SYSTEMS

An entrepreneurial health system in a highly industrialized country is best illustrated by that in the United States. Indeed, in 1990 there is probably no other country that belongs in this category, although Australia may have fitted into it 20 years before.

Health resources of all sorts are relatively abundant in the United States. Physicians are plentiful (about 220 per 100,000 population), and for each physician there are 15 or 20 associated health personnel—nurses, pharmacists, dentists, technicians, physical therapists, administrators. These personnel are prepared by universities, hospitals, and other training centers that are sponsored about half by units of government and half by nongovernment agencies. Within medicine, there is a high degree of specialization, so that only about 15 percent of doctors are generalists. Of all doctors serving ambulatory patients, about half are in group practice clinics (three or more working together). About two-thirds of hospital beds are in nongovernmental institutions, and 10 percent of the total are operated for profit.

The major health authority of the U.S. federal government is the Department of Health and Human Services, which promotes disease prevention and gives medical care to selected population groups. In the 50 states and 3,100 counties, there are local public health authorities engaged in environmental sanitation, communicable-disease control, preventive service for mothers and infants, and certain other functions. Voluntary health agencies, focusing on certain persons, diseases, or services, are especially numerous. The largest channel for providing health care, however, is the private market of thousands of independent medical practitioners, pharmacies, laboratories, and so on.

Economic support for the U.S. health system comes predominantly from private sources—for about 60 percent of the vast expenditures in 1987 of $2,200 per capita. Of these health funds spent in the private sector, about half are derived from voluntary insurance, sold by hundreds of commercial or nonprofit companies. The public sector of 40 percent is derived partly from social insurance (Social Security legislation) and partly from federal, state, and local tax revenues. Charity and industrial management contribute only a small fraction (under 5 percent) of health-system costs. As a share of gross national product (GNP), U.S. health expenditures consume 11.5 percent—the largest percentage of any country. Still, some 15 percent of the population are without adequate economic protection for health-care costs.

Since the U.S. health system is so pluralistic in structure and function, primary health care is not delivered in a uniform way. Most is provided by private practitioners, who are paid fees for each service rendered—whether the source of payment is private or public.

The largest governmentally sponsored programs of medical care are Medicare for the elderly and totally disabled and Medicaid for the poor. Under both of these programs doctors and other practitioners are paid by the fee-for-service method, administered with much elasticity. This applies to services in hospitals, which usually have "open" medical staffs, and to care of the ambulatory patient.

In spite of these highly entrepreneurial characteristics, the U.S. health system has been undergoing rapid changes. The long-term trend of economic support has been toward increased financing through collectivized mechanisms. The delivery of health service has also been subjected to various patterns of organization, so that teams of health personnel working in clinics, community health centers, and hospitals are becoming increasingly common. Various legislative strategies are being actively debated to achieve universal coverage for health services in the United States.

An entrepreneurial type of health system in a middle-income developing country is found in the Philippine Republic. Despite the general poverty of the national population (GNP per capita in 1986 was $590), of all health-related expenditures in 1980, 75 percent came from private sources. There are 76 provinces with locally elected governors, but the central Ministry of Health, like other ministries, has its own representatives in each province. The provincial health officers, and below them, district health officers, theoretically supervise MoH hospitals, but most of their work concerns conventional preventive public health services.

Major responsibility for financing medical care is vested in the Philippine Medical Care Commission, which is independent of the MoH. It administers a social insurance program, covering in 1980 about 28 percent of the population. Unlike policies in welfare-oriented health systems, these constitute *higher*-paid employees in public and private employment. The services are rendered by private physicians and private hospitals that are paid on a fee-for-service basis. When costs rose steeply in the late 1970s, the solution was not to reduce private fees but to increase cost sharing required from patients.

The output of physicians and nurses in the Philippines is quite high, but more than half of the new graduates leave the country. In 1984, therefore, there were in the country only 14.3 physicians per 100,000 population; more than half of these were settled in and around the national capital, with 22 percent of the people. There are 23 medical schools training physicians, but only three are governmental; the other 20 are small private schools run by private doctors as profit-making enterprises. Likewise, 87 percent of 132 nursing schools were privately owned and operated.

Of all Philippine physicians, 59 percent in 1981 were engaged entirely in private practice. Nearly all of the 41 percent in government employment also did private work part-time. Among dentists, 84 percent were wholly private. Hospitals are relatively abundant, with 1.8 beds per 1,000 people in 1981. Of the 1,600 facilities, however, 74 percent were private, with 55 percent of the total beds. Only affluent patients and some covered by the social insurance (who can afford the copayments) can use the private hospitals. Even the public hospitals make charges for drugs and diagnostic procedures, except to totally indigent patients. The 45 percent of beds in public hospitals are typically overcrowded, with frequent occupancy of one bed by two patients.

The Philippine health system had some 2,000 health centers for ambulatory service in 1982. While theoretically staffed by a doctor, nurse, and midwife, the health centers have many vacancies. The services offered are limited essentially to prevention, and patients coming for treatment (except for first aid) are usually sent to a private physician or a hospital outpatient department. The rate of health-center utilization is, therefore, very low.

The high percentage of private health expenditures has been noted. Considering personal household spending, a 1975 survey found that drugs and medical supplies accounted for 45 percent, private physicians and healers for 25 percent, and fees payable to hospitals and other facilities for 30 percent.

A low-income developing country of Africa, with entrepreneurial health-system policies, is Kenya. Its GNP per capita in 1986 was only $324, but its ruling Kenya African National Union (KANU) party has been committed to a policy of free private enterprise.

The seven provinces and, within these, 41 districts are each headed by a medical officer, who is appointed by the central government. Below the level of the district, planning in 1972 called for 254 "rural health units" (staffed entirely by auxiliary personnel), but by 1984, only 120 of these were in operation. The Kenyan government estimated that primary health care had been brought within reach of about 30 percent of the rural population. The Ministry of Local Government also has responsibilities for health in the country's four main cities.

Loosely linked to the MoH is a National Hospital Insurance Fund that insures about 12 percent of the population. As in the Philippines, it is the higher-paid employed or self-employed persons who must pay premiums, and there is no contribution from employers. The insurance fund is explicitly intended to increase the use of private hospitals or private beds in public hospitals.

There are many nongovernmental health agencies in Kenya, the most important religious missions from Europe and America. In 1981 these missions controlled about 25 percent of the hospital beds, while 46 percent were in government facilities and 29 percent were purely private. The mission hospitals got 24 percent of their operating costs from government grants, but 60 percent came from private-patient fees (sometimes through insurance).

Kenya's physicians numbered 10.5 per 100,000 population in 1981; of these, 53 percent were in the national capital, Nairobi, with 6 percent of the population, and 94 percent of the people had to depend on the remaining 47 percent of doctors. In 1982, at least 70 percent of all Kenyan physicians were entirely in private practice, and the 30 percent in government also practiced privately part-time.

It is not surprising, therefore, that a British study of health expenditures in Kenya in 1983–1984 found 49 percent from public sources and 51 percent from private. Household interviews revealed that 56 percent of the private expenditures came from a small proportion of families with high incomes. Also, 83 percent of the private spending came from the 15 percent who were city residents. The outcome of all these entrepreneurial policies as of 1986 is a life expectancy at birth of only 57 years, compared with 61 years in others countries of comparable income level (GNPs of $400 per capita or less).

WELFARE-ORIENTED HEALTH SYSTEMS

Many health systems of Western Europe are welfare-oriented, as are the systems of Canada, Japan, and Australia. The health system of the Federal Republic of Germany has mobilized economic support to make health service available to practically all its people for the longest period of time, so that it may well serve to illustrate this type in an industrialized country.

After many years of voluntary health-care insurance organizations among low-income workers. Germany enacted mandatory legislation for such insurance in 1883. The kinds of workers covered and the scope of health services provided were gradually broadened. The insurance is now carried by several hundred relatively small "sickness funds" that are regulated by government for costs, benefits, and methods of administration. The principal governmental responsibility for this social insurance is the Ministry of Labor and Social

Affairs in the central government and in each of the nine "länder" or provinces. Preventive public health work is done by the Ministry of Youth, Family Affairs, and Health working in local communities.

The education of physicians and other health personnel occurs in universities and schools sponsored entirely by units of government. Hospitals are also sponsored mainly (52.3 percent of beds in 1980) by units of government; of the nongovernmental hospital beds, two-thirds are under voluntary nonprofit agencies, and one-third are proprietary. The medical staffs of the proprietary hospitals are open to any qualified local physician, but in government and voluntary nonprofit facilities there are "closed" medical staffs of salaried physicians.

The payment of nonsalaried physicians for their services in Germany is a complex process, resulting from long historical developments. The sickness funds enter into contracts with associations of physicians, which are paid periodic per capita amounts according to each fund's membership. Then the medical association reviews and pays the fees charged by physicians. If in a quarter year the fees charged exceed the money available, less than the full amount of each fee may be paid; alternatively, certain doctors (suspected of over-servicing patients) may be underpaid. To safeguard the earnings of specialists in private practice, hospitals do not offer outpatient services, except for emergency cases.

The German pharmaceutical industry, largely an offshoot of the dye industry, is especially robust. Hundreds of new or slightly modified drugs are produced each year and dispensed by private pharmacies. The tragedy of Thalidomide—causing severely defective babies when taken by the pregnant women—occurred in West Germany in the 1960s and led to more regulatory drug legislation in Germany and many other countries. On the other hand, one must recognize that the principle of chemotherapy originated in 1912 in Germany (Paul Ehrlich and "Salvarsan"), and the sulfonamides were first synthesized by German chemists.

In contrast to the United States, the entire health system in Germany required expenditures of 8.2 percent of the gross domestic product (GDP) as of 1987. Of this amount, 77 percent was derived from programs under government, and only 23 percent came from the private sector. Most of the public funds came from the social insurance administered by the sickness funds. In spite of Germany's period of brutal fascism and the experience of defeat in two world wars, the German health system has continued to serve the great majority of the population well to the present.

The other welfare-oriented health systems of Western Europe are similar to the German in their use of many local insurance organizations to administer health-service financing. Each system, however, has certain unique characteristics. In France, for example, the patient must make payment for services directly to the physician and then seek reimbursement from his or her *"caisse de maladie"* according to a "nomenclature" (fees negotiated between the government and the medical association). Typically, the reimbursement is for 80 percent of the charges, so that the patient copays 20 percent. Administrative mechanisms in Belgium, the Netherlands, and Austria differ in other ways.

The welfare-oriented health systems of Australia and Canada are more fully under the umbrella of government, without use of intermediary insurance agencies. In Australia, there was no history of workers' insurance funds, so that health insurance is managed by a single national-government authority. In Canada, the key administrative bodies are the provincial governments, with partial funding by grants from the federal government. In both countries, funds come mainly from general revenues rather than earmarked employer-employee contributions to finance the programs. Most of the health services are still provided by private doctors, who are paid by negotiated fees, and hospitals are paid by prospective global budgets. In Australia, most hospitals are sponsored by local governments, and in Canada the majority is controlled by churches or other voluntary bodies.

Among developing countries, there are many with welfare-oriented health systems. At the middle-income level, many are in Latin America, where Social Security programs have been organized for varying proportions of the population. Peru, with a national population of about 20 million and a GNP per capita of $1,153 in 1986, may be taken as illustrative.

Since 1960, Peru has become rapidly urbanized, to 67 percent of its residents in 1984; this has meant a reduced dependence on traditional healers, or *curanderos*. It has also meant somewhat greater access of people to organized health programs that are strongest in the cities. In 1968, the Peruvian government was seized by a military coup that, paradoxically, brought about agrarian land reforms and nationalized certain industries. In 1976 another, more conservative military group seized power, but in 1980 a democratic civilian government was established with national elections.

The Peruvian Ministry of Health developed by 1985 a national network of 612 health centers and 1,700 health posts. Scores of charitable *"beneficencia"* hospitals were taken over by the MoH, so that 55.2 percent of the hospital beds (1.56 per 1,000 people) belong to the MoH. Along with the beds of other public agencies, government controls more than 80 percent of the total bed supply.

The country is divided into 17 health regions, and these into 57 health areas. The medical officers in charge of each jurisdiction, centrally appointed, are supposed to supervise all MoH services within their borders. The ambulatory-care facilities give general primary care, including treatment of common ailments, although preventive maternal and child health services are emphasized.

Like nearly all Latin American countries, Peru has a Social Security program providing medical care to 18.6 percent of the population. Unlike the Philippines or Germany, this social insurance program provides care in its own polyclinics and hospitals staffed by salaried medical and allied personnel. In 1975, the two previously separate social insurance programs for manual and white-collar workers are unified. However, any covered person, willing and able to make substantial copayments may consult private physicians and hospitals, and a small percentage does so.

Physicians in Peru numbered 17,500 in 1985, or 91.5 per 100,000 population. Some 70 percent of these work in government agencies but practice privately part-time, and 30 percent are wholly in private practice. There are seven medical schools, of which only one is private. Maldistribution of doctors is extreme, with 70 percent in 1985 located in Lima where 16 percent of the population resides. Among dentists, public employment is less common, and 72 percent are entirely private. Out-of-hospital drug consumption is high, and more than half of household health expenditures in 1984 went for self-prescribed drugs.

The welfare-oriented policies in the Peruvian health system are probably best reflected by overall health expenditures. In 1984, 66.5 percent of these came from government and 33.5 percent from private sources. The benefits of organized health services, in spite of general economic difficulties, are reflected in tuberculosis data. MoH reports indicated 225 cases per 100,000 population in 1962, and this rate was still 150 cases per 100,000 in 1983. Mortality, however, was 37.8 tuberculosis deaths per 100,000 in 1970 and declined to 17.6 deaths per 100,000 in 1984.

India is a low-income country with a welfare-oriented health system having characteristics quite different from those in Peru. This huge country of more than 800 million people had a GNP per capita of only $290 in 1986. Since it won independence from British rule in 1947, India has developed a national health system with thousands of publicly financed and publicly operated health facilities.

Continued from colonial times, India has 31 states and union territories that carry major health service responsibilities. In each of these jurisdictions there is a Ministry of Health and Family Welfare responsible for personal and environmental health services. Within the states and territories there are 408 districts, each containing an average of 2 million people and headed by a Medical Officer of Health. Two-thirds of MOHFW financing comes from the state level and one-third from the national level, the latter mainly for family planning to control population growth.

In every district of India there is a public hospital and several "primary health centers"—8,000 of them in 1988. These are ideally staffed by one or two physicians and allied health staff, but there are many medical vacancies. Around the primary health centers are more than 100,000 subcenters, staffed entirely by briefly trained auxiliary personnel. Because of the varying economic levels of the states, there are great differences in the amplitude of these resources. Peripheral to the subcenters, there are "community health volunteers," trained for a few weeks to encourage sound health practices in the villages.

Although India is only slightly industrialized, it has a Social Security program covering employees of private firms and their dependents, in 1987, 28 million people, or 3.5 percent of the population, entitled to medical care through specially organized facilities or regular MoHFW resources under contract. In large cities insured persons may be served by private general practitioners paid by capitation. There is a similar social insurance scheme, with organized medical services, for central-government employees.

India has 125 medical schools linked to universities that are almost entirely public and supervised by the Ministry of Education of each state. There are hundreds of voluntary health agencies, many tied to foreign religious missions. The latter operate small hospitals with 26 percent of the national stock of hospital beds.

Of all modern physicians in India, 41 percent work for government health agencies, 12 percent for nongovernmental but organized health programs, and 47 percent entirely in private practice. Altogether, in 1987 there were about 325,000 modern physicians, or 41 per 100,000 population. A much greater number of traditional doctors, however, were almost entirely in private practice throughout India; this included some 400,000 Ayurvedic practitioners (many trained in government-run colleges) and 150,000 homeopathic doctors. Since the late 1970s, the government of India has stressed the training of multipurpose auxiliary health personnel.

Health centers and subcenters for ambulatory care have been noted, and these are almost entirely governmental. Of the 550,000 hospital beds (0.71 per 1,000 people), 70 percent were controlled by central or state governments, another 4.6 percent by local authorities. Regarding another resource, pharmaceutical products, India has been successful in converting multinational into domestic production. In terms of the value of finished drug products, by 1972 government enterprises were producing 34 percent, private but domestically owned enterprises were producing 39 percent, and only 27 percent of finished products were produced by firms under foreign ownership.

In the early 1980s, total Indian health expenditures amounted to only 3 percent of the GNP. Of this, a study in 1970 found 84 percent from private sources, and it is likely that the private sector stills accounts for two-thirds of the total (as in neighboring Pakistan). If so, one-third of spending by the public sector constitutes an improvement in equity. For the fight against certain diseases, the national and state MoHFWs in India conduct special campaigns—previously run vertically from the top, but now decentralized. These include the reduction of infant diarrhea (oral rehydration therapy), malaria control, tuberculosis control, the WHO "expanded program of immunization," leprosy control, and family planning. Improvements have resulted from all these campaigns. Life expectancy at birth in India has increased from 44 in 1960 to 59 in 1987. Even the crude birthrate, contributing to India's huge population, has declined between these years from 42 to 32 per 1,000 population.

COMPREHENSIVE HEALTH SYSTEMS

In several countries, national health systems that were welfare-oriented for some years underwent further political development after World War II and became comprehensive. This has meant that 100 percent of the national population has become entitled to complete health service, and the financial support has shifted almost entirely to general tax revenues. Larger proportions of doctors and other health personnel have come to work in organized frameworks on salary. Almost all health facilities have come under the direct control of government.

Great Britain adopted this comprehensive type of health system soon after World War II pursuant to planning during the war. The Scandinavian countries did likewise in the 1950s. Italy enacted "national health service" legislation in the 1970s, and somewhat less sweepingly this was done in Greece and Spain. The British National Health Service (NHS) has had worldwide impacts, so this may illustrate the comprehensive health system.

Limited insurance for general-practitioner services and drugs had covered low-wage manual workers in Great Britain since 1911. With the 1946 legislation, this program was expanded to provide all ambulatory-treatment services and to become the first pillar of the NHS. Because of the war, British hospitals had been organized into regional groups, and these, headed by regional hospital boards, became the second organizational pillar. Local public health authorities, along with visiting nurse and ambulance services, became the third pillar. Finally, a special administrative channel was reserved for teaching hospitals affiliated with medical schools. In this three- or four-part administrative structure, policies on professional remuneration varied pragmatically. General practitioners were paid by capitation, according to the persons enrolled with each one. Dentists were paid by fees for each unit of service. Specialists (or consultants), who were hospital-based, were employed by the regional boards and paid by salaries.

In 1974, the British NHS was reorganized to achieve greater administrative integration. After a preliminary period, all health services were placed under unified management in some 200 health districts. At this level, a well-trained specialist in management was supported by a specialist in community medicine (including epidemiology). The regional hospital boards were converted into regional health boards and became the conduits for money from the central government. At all levels there were "community health councils" composed of leading consumers and providers for advisory purposes.

Popular opinion in Great Britain has been highly favorable toward the NHS, although there are complaints about long waiting lists for elective (nonemergency) surgery in hospitals. The explanation of these delays is fundamentally that the resources provided by government for this large comprehensive health system are inadequate. In 1987, when the United States was spending 11.2 percent of gross domestic product on health and Sweden was spending 9.0 percent, Great Britain was spending only 6.1 percent of its smaller overall GDP. Of this expenditure, 87 percent came from government and 13 percent from the private sector. (In 1975, however, only 9 percent of British health expenditures had been private, and Conservative government policy has encouraged greater private spending.)

The development of comprehensive health systems in the Scandinavian countries was more gradual. The local workers' health insurance funds were simply converted into branch offices of the national government, and services became available to everyone. The demand for health services in Norway and Sweden does not seem to be as high as in Great Britain, yet both human and physical resources are relatively greater. In Sweden, for example, the health spending in 1987 amounted to 9 percent of GDP, of which 91 percent came from public sources and 9 percent from private. This was an increase from 8 percent of GDP in 1975, of which (in contrast to Britain) 10 percent, a slightly greater fraction, had previously come from private sources. The Swedish government, in other words, has responded to rising demand by strengthening the public sector.

Among developing countries, there are very few that have achieved comprehensive health systems that have entitled 100 percent of their populations to complete health services. One of middle-income level is Costa Rica, which in 1948 abolished its military establishment and gradually extended its Social Security coverage for medical care to everyone. Another country of very low-income level (GNP per capita of $400 in 1986) is Sri Lanka, a tropical island south of India.

In 1986, Sri Lanka had 16 million people, with the same sort of vast disparities in family wealth as most developing countries. The richest 20 percent of households earned 50 percent of the total income, while the poorest 20 percent earned only 6 percent. Yet the government health services made available to all these people are remarkably complete. For governance, the country is divided into 25 districts, each headed by a centrally appointed medical officer. Within each district, there are about 10 divisions, averaging 60,000 people, with a medically staffed "divisional health center." More peripherally, there are "subdivisional health centers," staffed wholly by auxiliary personnel, including "assistant medical practitioners" with two years of training in primary health care. Voluntary health agencies are also strong in Sri Lanka, especially the Red Cross, the Cancer Society, and the Family Planning Association.

The supply of modern physicians in Sri Lanka is quite modest—13.4 per 100,000 in 1981—because many are Tamils, who faced ethnic discrimination and therefore emigrated. The stock of Ayurvedic practitioners is three times as great, and these are virtually all in private practice. Government health labor needs in Sri Lanka are met largely by auxiliary personnel.

Nutrition policy in Sri Lanka has been a major factor contributing to health. Soon after independence in 1947, a weekly ration of rice was provided free to every family; even when this was altered in the 1970s, it was continued for very poor families, along with free lunches for all schoolchildren. General education has also had high priority in Sri Lanka. Nearly all girls and boys go to primary school, and in 1985 adult literacy was 91 percent for men; 83 percent for women.

The Sri Lankan Ministry of Health in the mid-1980s estimated that

93 percent of the population were readily accessible to health services. Because of the shortage of modern physicians, Ayurvedic practitioners are consulted extensively; many of these make use of penicillin and other scientific drugs.

Because of its closeness to India and its cultural similarities, Sri Lanka's health record has often been compared to India's. In 1985, when India's infant mortality rate was 105 per 1,000 live biths, the rate in Sri Lanka was 36 per 1,000. In 1987, life expectancy at birth in India was 59; in Sri Lanka, 71. Strong programs of nutrition and educatiaon have doubtless contributed importantly to these achievements, but the comprehensive health system has surely played a substantial part.

SOCIALIST HEALTH SYSTEMS

In countries that have had a revolution to install a socialist economic order, the health systems have become socialist in structure and function. This has meant that practically all physical and human resources have been taken over by government and health services have theoretically become available to everyone. In 1989 and 1990, certain basic changes were brought about in these socialist economies, but conditions will be described as they were shortly before this. (The patterns to be adopted after 1990 were far from clear.)

After the Russian Revolution of 1917, the Soviet Union became the first country with a socialist health system. The changes did not occur overnight but were essentially completed by 1937. By then, virtually all doctors, nurses, and other health personnel had become public employees, and all hospitals and other health facilities were taken over by government. The private pharmaceutical industry was nationalized; medical schools were removed from the universities and put under the Ministry of Health as academic institutes. Health-science research was carried out in other special institutes, also under the Ministry of Health.

All services were free to every Soviet resident, except drugs, which had to be purchased in government pharmacies. Certain lifesaving compounds, however, and all drugs for certain persons (military veterans or pensioners) were free. To provide accessible ambulatory care, hundreds of polyclinics—staffed by generalists, pediatricians, gynecologists, and others—were established in the cities, and hundreds of small health centers were constructed in rural areas. The Soviet *feldsher*, trained since the nineteenth century, was one of the world's earliest forms of medical assistant, serving mostly in rural areas where physicians were too few.

The Soviet health system has turned out enormous numbers of physicians, so that in 1986 there were 430 per 100,000 population. Nurses, midwives, and feldshers were also plentiful, but technicians were relatively less numerous than in other industrialized countries. Diagnostic and therapeutic equipment in hospitals was generally less developed than in Western European countries, a deficiency that President Gorbachev's *perestroika* (restructuring) was expected to correct. Certain exceptionally well-equipped and well-staffed hospitals and polyclinics, however, were established to serve high Communist party officials. Such "preferred care" is provided for "important persons" in most national health systems, but in egalitarian socialist societies it has caused much popular resentment.

Since about 1960, private out-of-hospital health service has expanded slightly in the Soviet Union for people who can afford to pay private fees. These "paying polyclinics" are staffed by hospital-based specialists, who may work in them a limited number of hours per week. As a general backup for all polyclinics and hospitals, all large Soviet cities have well-developed emergency services staffed by physicians and feldshers, and equipped with modern ambulances. Calls to a central telephone exchange lead to the dispatch of ambulances from various locations in large metropolitan areas.

The health of the population in the Soviet Union improved markedly after the 1917 Revolution for about 50 years. The infant mortality rate declined, and the life expectancy at birth increased significantly. Then in the 1970s these indexes changed, and health conditions clearly deteriorated. Various explanations were offered, but most important seemed to be the cold war and the vast military expenditures it entailed. The funds remaining for health services were seriously inadequate. Soviet health-system expenditures in the 1970s and 1980s were less than 4 percent of national wealth (as calculated by economists from international agencies). This was much lower than in any Western industrialized country and far below the health needs. As part of perestroika, health expenditures were expected to increase, but the effects of this would take time to see. In the other socialist countries of Eastern Europe (Poland, Hungary, etc.), the health systems were modeled after that of the Soviet Union, and the transformations toward a free-market pattern were occurring somewhat earlier in the 1980s.

Cuba is a middle-income developing country that had a social revolution in 1959 and then introduced a thoroughly socialist health system. The Cuban population is 10 million, and its GNP per capita in 1986 was just under $2,000. The adult literacy attained by 1984 was 96 percent.

As in other socialist countries, practically all responsibility for health services is under the Ministry of Public Health (MINSAP in the Spanish acronym). After several changes since 1959, the country has become divided into 14 health provinces, each headed by a centrally appointed medical officer. Within the provinces are 169 urban or rural municipalities, which elect local assemblies, and these appoint municipal medical officers. Voluntary agencies are limited to "mass organizations" of women, farmers, workers, and youth, who help out in health campaigns. There is virtually no market for private medical care, either modern or traditional.

Health education was greatly expanded after the Cuban revolution to compensate for the 33 to 50 percent of former physicians, dentists, and pharmacists who left the country. By 1968, medical schools had been increased from one to four, and by 1982 there were 17,000 active physicians (about half, women), for a ratio of 170 per 100,000 population. Schools for nurses, dentists, and technicians were also expanded, but Cuba rejected the idea of the feldsher or general medical assistant. Leaders said that a revolutionary health system had no place for "second-class doctors" nor for other types of "community health workers." Cuba has not even trained professional midwives; all childbirths are attended by physicians in hospitals.

Physical facilities were also greatly expanded in Cuba after the revolution. By 1982 there were 5.3 hospital beds per 1,000 people, and their geographic distribution was largely equalized. Before 1959, metropolitan Havana had 62 percent of the beds, and the much larger rural population had 38 percent; in 1982, Havana had 39 percent of the beds, and 61 percent were in the rest of the country.

The most important physical structures in the Cuban health system are the 425 polyclinics, each serving about 25,000 people for general ambulatory care, preventive and curative. For each 5,000 people there is normally a team of four physicians (internist, pediatrician, obstetrician-gynecologist, and dentist), so that there would ideally be five such teams in each polyclinic. For preventive attention to cases with chronic disorders, patients are called back periodically for checkups and counseling (a practice called dispensarization).

Since 1983, Cuba has been placing "family practitioners" at posts around the polyclinic to provide general primary health care to only 600–700 persons. These generalists are then backed up by the polyclinic medical teams. Cuba's attitude on family planning is not aggressive since there is a need for more population; contraceptive advice and supplies, however, are freely available on request.

As a result of its overall socioeconomic policies and its health system, Cuba has attained the best health record of any country in Latin America, including several of much greater per capita wealth. The infant mortality rate was reduced to 15.0 per 1,000 live births by 1986. Life expectancy at birth had been 61.8 years in 1960, and by 1982 it was extended to 73.5 years.

A socialist country that had a social revolution in 1949 is the People's Republic of China, with more than 1 billion people and a very complex social history. It is not easy to summarize China's health system, but the highlights may be given. In spite of its socialist ideology, China's overall income level is so low that government-financed health services for all have not yet been achieved.

Having passed through several major periods of political change since the earlier bourgeois revolution of 1911, by 1986, China had a ratio of 57 modern physicians per 100,000 population. There were also 32 traditional Chinese practitioners per 100,000, and although official policy called for their integration into the government health services, the great majority were in private practice. In addition, there are thousands of assistant doctors (45 per 100,000 people) trained in "secondary medical schools" for three years—not to be confused with "barefoot doctors." These secondary medical schools also train nurses, technicians, and pharmacy assistants. The "barefoot doctor" was a peasant trained for only a few months, principally during the period of the Cultural Revolution (1965–1975). At their peak there were 1 million of these auxiliaries, and after the death of Chairman Mao Tse-tung in 1976, they were upgraded to "village doctors," numbering 1,245,000 in 1989.

Hospital supply was also vastly expanded in socialist China. By 1985, there were hospitals in all 2,300 counties and a ratio of 2.1 beds per 1,000 population. Formerly the counties were organized into 27,000 "communes" for local agricultural and other production, but these have been converted to "townships." Each township and municipal district has health centers for general primary health care. In 1986, there were 48,100 such facilities, each serving an average of 22,000 people. In the cities, these were usually staffed by physicians, both Western and traditional; in small towns, they would have only assistant doctors of both types and allied health personnel. Finally, in the villages, there are small health stations staffed with village doctors and aides, numbering some 126,000 structures in 1985.

Through deliberate planning, China has developed 800 pharmaceutical plants that produce some 3,000 modern drug compounds;

in addition, it has 480 plants for manufacture of traditional drugs. These drugs are distributed through some 360 pharmaceutical warehouses in the provinces to hospitals, health centers, and some 20,000 local pharmacies. The latter were originally under the Ministry of Public Health, but since 1980, many have become private.

The central MoPH establishes general policies, but most responsibility is carried by corresponding agencies in each of the 21 mainland provinces, 5 autonomous regions, and 3 centrally administered municipalities. Some 90 percent of financial support must come from each province. Every county also has a Bureau of Public Health, headed by a modern physician, but below this level, health-service management is simply by the health-center staff.

To help meet the costs of medical care in hospitals and health centers, several forms of health insurance have been developed: (1) for central-government employees (but not dependents), the Ministry of Finance; (2) for workers in national or provincial enterprises, including dependents, each enterprise, supervised by the Ministry of Labor; (3) for workers in enterprises of the counties, municipalities, and townships, with some protection of dependents; and (4) for farm families, through local health cooperatives. The coverage of dependent costs in these insurance programs is usually 50 percent of the official fees. According to a World Bank analysis, in 1987 all these forms of insurance accounted for 50 percent of health-system expenditures; overall government revenues at all levels contributed 19 percent, and private individuals had to pay fees amounting to 32 percent. Health insurance covers about 40 percent of the national population with some protection.

Public health campaigns against malaria, schistosomiasis, tuberculosis, and other diseases are carried out by the provincial ministries of public health. Research, education, construction of facilities, and management of all hospitals and health centers are all functions of government. It is the large recurrent expenditures for personal medical care in China that must be paid for privately or through health insurance. Also, since 1980, a growing proportion of modern physicians and even village doctors have undertaken private practice.

Family planning has been a major part of China's social policy since 1968. By 1987, the crude birthrate was reduced to 20 per 1,000 people. Health achievements have likewise been impressive. Infant mortality was reduced from 150 deaths per 1,000 live births in 1960 to 33 per 1,000 in 1987. Life expectancy at birth over the same period was extended from 47 to 70. Even though serious inequities persist in the operation of China's health system, its achievements have won worldwide admiration.

GENERAL TRENDS

In all four types of national health system, in industrialized as well as developing countries, certain general trends have been evident over the last 50 years. The resources, both human and physical, have been greatly expanded. As more people have survived to the older age groups and as educational levels have improved, the demands for personal health care everywhere have risen. Every country has responded by developing larger resources and new kinds of health personnel. Pharmaceutical products have also increased in quantity, variety, and effectiveness.

The organization of health systems, largely under government, has increased and grown more complex. Agencies, public and private, have multiplied, and in general the strength and scope of ministries of health have been enhanced. Public health authorities have grown at various jurisdictional levels, local and provincial as well as national. Nongovernmental voluntary agencies have also grown to promote health efforts regarding certain persons, disorders, or services.

The management of national health systems has become generally more sophisticated as the interests of more groups of health-care providers and consumers become defined. Administrators are trained, record systems are formulated, consumers are given a stronger voice, and decision making has become a more democratic process. To limit abuses in the private market, regulatory powers have been extended. More and more aspects of health are being subjected to legislative intervention—from reducing the sale of harmful tobacco products to the mobilization of funds for supporting the costs of prevention and treatment.

As a share of national wealth, the money devoted to health systems has increased steadily, except perhaps in the European socialist countries. It has grown in both public and private sectors, although in all but a few countries more rapidly in the public sector. Of all the health services, those in hospitals have absorbed the most rapidly expanding proportion to provide the benefits of advanced technology to an aging population with chronic diseases. With the objective of meeting the health needs of more people, rural and urban, the World Health Organization has stressed everywhere a higher priority for primary health care.

In the delivery of health care, the key concept has become teamwork. The importance of this has long been recognized in hospitals, and it is now appreciated in ambulatory care. The socialist countries first demonstrated the value of polyclinics and health centers to provide integrated preventive-curative services to general populations, and all countries with other types of health systems have to some extent acted likewise. There is a generally increased application of these organized frameworks, from the entrepreneurial to the socialist health systems.

These developments in all components of national health systems add up to the attainment of greater health-care equity in the world. In the words of the Constitution of the World Health Organization, it has long been agreed that "The enjoyment of the highest attainable standard of health is one of the fundamental rights of every human being, without distinction of race, religion, political belief, economic or social condition."

Implementation of this ideal may lie in the future, but the developments in national health systems over the last half century give grounds for confidence about its ultimate achievement.

REFERENCES

Bosch, Paul F. *Textbook of International Health*. New York: Oxford University Press, 1990.

Elling, Ray H. *Cross-National Study of Health Systems*. New Brunswick, NJ: Transaction Books, 1980.

Organization for Economic Cooperation and Development. *Health Care Systems in Transition*. Paris: OECD, 1990.

Pannenborg, P. O., et al., (eds.) *Reorienting Health Services: Application of a Systems Approach*. New York: Plenum Press, 1984.

Raffel, Marshall W., (ed.) *Comparative Health Systems: Descriptive Analyses of Fourteen National Health Systems*. University Park, PA: Pennsylvania State University Press, 1984.

Roemer, Milton I. *National Health Systems of the World*. New York: Oxford University Press, 1991.

Saltman, Richard B., ed. *The International Headbook of Health-Care Systems*. Westport, CT: Greenwood Press, 1988.

Critical Reports/ Analyses of the U.S. Health Care Delivery System, 1927–1983

Business Week. "The $60-Billion Crisis over Medical Care," Special reprint, January 17, 1970.

Citizen's Board of Inquiry into Health Services for Americans. *Heal Yourself* (report). Washington, D.C.: Citizen's Board of Inquiry into Health Services for Americans, 1971.

Ehrenreich, B., & Ehrenreich, J. *The American Health Empire: Power, Profits, and Politics.* New York: Vintage Books, 1971.

Harper's Magazine. "The Crisis in American Medicine," October 1960, p. 123.

Healthline. "American Health Care: A System in Crisis," October 1983, p. 7.

Health Task Force of the Urban Coalition. *Rx for Action* (report). Washington, D.C.; 1969.

Jonas, S. *Medical Mystery: The Training of Doctors in the United States.* New York: W. W. Norton, 1979.

Kennedy, E. M. *In Critical Condition.* New York: Simon and Schuster, 1972.

Knowles, J. H. ed. *Doing Better and Feeling Worse.* New York: W. W. Norton, 1977.

Moskin, J. R. "The Challenge to Our Doctors." *Look,* November 3, 1964, p. 26.

National Commission on Community Health Services. *Health Is a Community Affair.* Cambridge, MA: Harvard University Press. 1966.

Ribicoff, A., Danaceau, P. *The American Medical Machine.* New York: Saturday Review Press, 1972.

Schorr, D. *Don't Get Sick in America.* Nashville, TN: Aurora Publishers, 1970.

Silver, G.A. *A Spy in the House of Medicine.* Germantown, MD: Aspen Systems, 1976.

Sidel, V. W., & Sidel, R. *A Healthy State* (revised and updated). New York: Pantheon Books, 1983.

Somers, A. R., & Somers, H. M. *Health and Health Care.* Germantown, MD: Aspen Systems, 1977.

Further, in a review of the Ehrenreich & Ehrenreich book, *The American Health Empire: Power, Profits, and Politics* (cited above), which appeared in the *International Journal of Health Services, 2,* 119, 1972, Dr. Milton Roemer listed a series of other reports going back many years. He said (p. 119):

> Every few years, more recently in the last decade, there appears a book analyzing the serious defects of health care in America. In 1927, Harry H. Moore produced *American Medicine and the People's Health,* in the 1930's were the magnificent 27 volumes of the Committee on the Costs of Medical Care, in 1939 there was James Rorty's *American Medicine Mobilizes,* and in 1940 Hugh Cabot's *The Patient Dilemma.* After World War II, Carl Malmberg wrote *140 Million Patients* in 1947, Michael Davis wrote *Medical Care for Tomorrow* in 1955, and Richard Carter wrote *The Doctor Business* in 1958. In 1965 there was Selig Greenberg's excellent *The Troubled Calling: Crisis in the Medical Establishment.* The year after Medicare, 1966, saw two critical outputs: *The American Health Scandal* by Raul Tunley and *The Doctors* by Martin L. Gross. In 1967 there was Fred J. Cook's *Plot Against the Patient* and in 1970 Ed Cray's *In Failing Health.*

Guide to Sources

Part A of this guide contains descriptions of the major health and health-services data sources for the United States: who publishes them, how frequently they are published as of 1991, from whom they may be ordered, and what categories of data they contain. Also, in appendix I of the annual *Health United States* (DHHS Pub. No. [PHS] [year of publication]-1232) you can find very useful detailed descriptions of all the common health and health-services data sources, private and government. Appendix I of the *Statistical Abstract* (year of publication) also contains an extensive listing of sources of "Health and Medical Care" data. The American Hospital Association's *Guide Issue* (year of publication) contains a comprehensive listing of "Health Organizations, Agencies, Providers, Alliances and Networks" (Part D), from which much data can be obtained.

In Part B of this guide you will a listing of commonly sought-after categories of data and the publications from the list in Part A in which you can find them, as well as certain other sources.

PART A

1. *Statistical Abstract of the United States.* Published annually by the Bureau of the Census, U.S. Department of Commerce, Washington, D.C.,* the *Statistical Abstract* reproduces a vast selection of tables containing information from many different government agencies. They are accumulated under the following headings: Population; Vital Statistics; Health and Nutrition; Education; Law Enforcement, Courts, and Prisons; Geography and Environment; Parks, Recreation and Travel; Elections; Federal Government Finances and Employment; State and Local Government Finances and Employment; Federal Government Finances and Employment; National Defense

and Veterans' Affairs; Social Insurance and Human Services; Labor Force, Employment, and Earnings; Income, Expenditures, and Wealth; Prices; Banking, Finance, and Insurance; Business Enterprise; Communications; Energy; Science; Transportation—Land; Transportation—Air and Water; Agriculture; Forests and Fisheries; Mining and Mineral Products; Construction and Housing; Manufactures; Domestic Trade and Services; Foreign Commerce and Aid; Outlying Areas; and Comparative International Statistics. The *Abstract*'s large "Guide to Sources" covers many categories of data, and also lists some state and international data sources.

2. *U.S. Census of Population.* The Bureau of the Census is part of the U.S. Department of Commerce, Washington, D.C. 20233. The Constitution requires that a census be taken every 10 years, at the beginning of each decade. The original purpose was to apportion seats in the House of Representatives and thus in the Electoral College. In modern times, in addition to the simple counts, a great deal of demographic data is collected by the Census Bureau. Hardcover compendia of decennial national census data are published periodically. Also available are special analyses for a wide variety of geographical subdivisions of the country. Many reports on the decennial censuses are published by the Census Bureau, but a good place to begin is in Section I of the *Statistical Abstract*.

3. *Current Population Reports.* In addition to reports from the decennial censuses, the Census Bureau publishes seven series of reports on a continuing basis. These include estimates, projections, sample counts, and special studies of selected segments of the population. The seven series each have a P number: P-20, Population Characteristics; P-23, Special Studies; P-25, Population Estimates and Projections; P-26, Federal-State Cooperative Program for Population Estimates; P-27, Farm Population; P-28, Special Censuses; and P-60, Consumer Income. information on the content of each series is of course available from the Census Bureau. Subscriptions are not available for individual series but must be taken in two sets; however, single copies of reports from all series except P-28 may be ordered from the USGPO.

4. *Monthly Vital Statistics Report (MVSR).* MVSR is published by the National Center for Health Statistics, Centers for Disease Control, Department of Health and Human Services, 6525 Belcrest Road, Hyattsville, MD 20782. It has several sections. *Provisional Statistics,*

---

*Almost all U.S. government publications are to be purchased from the Superintendent of Documents, United States Government Printing Office (USGPO), Washington, D.C. 20402, rather than directly from the agency producing them.

published monthly, contains the most recent data for the traditional "vital statistics," deaths, births, marriages, and divorces. There is also a series of supplements, which appear on a semiregular basis and contain provisional final annual summaries of vital statistics plus technical information on methodology. In the *MVSR* there are also special reports that appear periodically. *MVSR* may be ordered by annual subscription.

5. *Vital Statistics of the United States.* This is the annual report of the National Center for Health Statistics (NCHS) concerning vital statistics. The address of the NCHS is given under *MVSR*, item 4 of this list.

6. *Vital and Health Statistics.* This publication of the NCHS appears periodically. There are 13 series, not numbered consecutively, most of which report data from ongoing studies and surveys that the NCHS has carried out. Several series have been dormant for some time. The publication of some data shifts periodically between *Vital and Health Statistics* and *Monthly Vital Statistics Report*. In the late 1970s, a new publication appeared: *Advance Data from Vital and Health Statistics. Advance Data* presents results from various ongoing NCHS surveys. The NCHS periodically publishes catalogs of their publications.

The 14 series in *Vital and Health Statistics* are as follows;

Series 1.   Programs and Collection Procedures
Series 2.   Data Evaluation and Methods Research
Series 3.   Analytical Studies (primarily of mortality, stressing international comparisons)
Series 4.   Documents and Committee Reports
Series 10.   Data from the Health Interview Survey (containing patient-perspective health, illness, and health-services utilization data)
Series 11.   Data from the Health Examination Survey and the Health and Nutrition Examination Survey
Series 12.   Data from the Health Records Survey (reports data from two studies of nursing homes carried out in the 1960s)
Series 13.   Data on Health Resources Utilization (includes hospitals, nursing homes, and ambulatory care services)
Series 14.   Data on Health Resources: Manpower and Facilities (health resources data appear also in *Health, United States* (see below)
Series 15.   Data from Special Surveys

Series 20.   Data on Mortality (reports of time-trends analyses
                for the United States)
Series 21.   Data on Natality, Marriage, and Divorce
Series 22.   Data from the National Natality and Mortality
                Surveys (different from Series 21 in that special
                studies are reported)
Series 23.   Data from the National Survey of Family Growth

7. *Morbidity and Mortality Weekly Report (MMWR).* This is a regular publication of the Center for Disease Control (CDC) of the USDHHS and is available on an annual subscription basis from the CDC, Atlanta, GA 30333. Following a large subscription price increase in 1982, *MMWR,* in the public domain, has been mass-photocopied and circulated at cost by several organizations including the Massachusetts Medical Society, c/o the *New England Journal of Medicine,* 10 Shattuck St., Boston, MA 02115. In the past, it has been concerned primarily with the communicable diseases for which reporting is required by law. Most of the diseases covered are no longer of much importance in the United States, and for many of them, the reporting rates are poor. Nevertheless, it provides an important perspective on communicable disease in the United States. Of course, with the advent of AIDS and the resurgence of the venereal diseases, communicable disease reporting has taken on new significance.

Each week, case reports of specific outbreaks of communicable diseases are reported; there are also occasional international notes, status reports on communicable disease control programs, and statements of official U.S. Public Health Service positions on various issues in communicable disease control. In recent years *MMWR* has acquired a broader preview, reporting on CDC, NIOSH, and USPHS activities in chronic disease control. Its value has increased significantly.

8. *Health United States.* The first edition of this work was published in 1976 under the title *Health, United States, 1975.* Now produced by the National Center for Health Statistics, it has appeared annually since then. In earlier issues, there were several review articles on "selected health topics," but this feature was eliminated in the mid-1980s in favor of a section of "Highlights" and a "Chartbook" section featuring commentary and charts on important conditions. In the body of the text data are grouped under Health Status and Determinants, Utilization of Health Resources, Health Care Resources, and Health Care Expenditures. There is also contains a useful appendix, Sources and Limitations of Data, and as a Glossary. *Health U.S.* is a boon to students and researchers in health-care delivery because it

provides one-stop shopping for most important health and health care data.

9. *American Hospital Association Guide to the Health Care Field.* This two-part publication of the American Hospital Association, 840 North Lake Shore Drive, Chicago IL 60611-2431, appears in August of each year. The first part, the *Guide to the Health Care Field*, contains a listing of almost every hospital in the United States by location and gives basic data on size, type, ownership, and facilities, as well as a great deal of information on the AHA and the hospital supply industry. The second part, *Hospital Statistics,* contains a much summary utilization and financial data on U.S. hospitals, by many different cross-tabulations. Some of the data are presented historically. The two parts together contain the most detailed available data on hospitals in the United States.

10. *Health Care Financing Review* is a quarterly published by the Health Care Financing Administration (HCFA). It contains many statistical reports, especially on health-care expenditures, and reports of special studies. HCFA publications are available from the USGPO.

11. "AAMC Data Reports" appear periodically in the journal *Academic Medicine* published by the Association of American Medical Colleges, 1 DuPont Circle, Washington, DC 20036. Together with the annual issue of the *Journal of the American Medical Association* on medical education, the "Data Reports" provide the principal source of data on medical education in the United States: schools, faculty, curricula, admissions, students, and the like.

12. *The American Medical Association.* Located at 535 North Dearborn Street, Chicago, IL 60610, the AMA produces a variety of useful data on the physician work force from its own files. The AMA regularly publishes a catalog of its publications. Other major professional organizations are good sources of data on their own members.

B. CATEGORIES OF DATA: SOURCES

(Where applicable, the number in parentheses following the title of a publication refers to its listing in Part A, above.)

1. Population Data
   a. *Statistical Abstract of the United States,* Section 1, (1).
   b. *U.S. Census of Population* (2).
   c. *Current Population Reports* (3).

    d. State and local governments. Some state and local governments, and/or state and local independent planning agencies, use detailed Census Bureau data on their local areas, which the bureau does not routinely publish, to produce very detailed compendia of local and/or state census data. Local inquiries must be made to determine if such information is available for a particular area.

    e. Utility companies. In many parts of the country, utility companies publish on a regular periodic basis estimates of population changes since the most recent census. They also often add other information, particularly concerning economic growth. Local inquiries should be made.

    f. *Health, United States* (8). Some population data are presented under "Health Status and Determinants."

2. *Vital Statistics*

    a. *Monthly Vital Statistics Report* (4).

    b. *Vital Statistics of the United States* (5).

    c. *Vital and Health Statistics* (6).

    d. Life Tables. These indicators, based on mortality data, are published independently and periodically by the National Center for Health Statistics.

    e. *Statistical Abstract of the United States* (1). Selected vital statistics appear annually in Section 2, "Vital Statistics."

    f. Health Departments. Some state and local health departments publish compendia of vital statistics for their jurisdictions.

    h. *Health, United States* (8). Some vital health data are presented under "Health Status and Determinants."

3. *Morbidity*

    a. *Vital and Health Statistics* (6). A wide variety of morbidity data from many different sources are published periodically in Series 10, 11, 12, and 13.

    b. *Advance Data* (6). A variety of morbidity data, some of which also appear in *Vital and Health Statistics*, are published on an irregular basis. They include data from the National Ambulatory Medical Care Survey, the Health and Nutrition Examination Survey, and the Hospital Discharge Survey.

    c. *Morbidity and Mortality Weekly Report* (7).

    d. *Statistical Abstract of the United States* (1). Selected morbidity statistics appear annually in Section 2, "Vital Statistics," and in Section 3, "Health and Nutrition."

    e. Health Departments. State and local health departments sometimes publish morbidity surveys for their jurisdictions.

f. *Health, United States* (8). Some morbidity data are presented under "Health Status and Determinants."

4. *Utilization of Health Services*
   a. *Vital and Health Statistics* (6). Series 10 presents patient-perspective data from the *Health Interview Survey*. Provider-perspective data are provided from the *National Ambulatory Medical Care Survey* (Series 2) and the *Hospital Discharge Survey* (Series 13). Some of these data also appear in *Advance Data*.
   b. *Guide to the Health Care Field and Hospital Statistics* (9).
   c. *Health, United States* (8). Patient- and provider-perspective utilization data are presented under "Utilization of Health Resources."
   d. American Medical Association (12). Various publications present provider-perspective utilization data.

5. *Institutions*
   a. *Statistical Abstract of the United States* (1). Basic data on health-care institution are contained in Section 3.
   b. *Vital and Health Statistics* (6). Data on institutions appear in Series 12, 13, and 14.
   c. *Health, United States* (8). Under "Utilization of Health Resources."
   d. *Guide to the Health Care Field and Hospital Statistics* (9).

6. *Health Personnel*
   a. *Statistical Abstract of the United States* (1). Section 3.
   b. *Vital and Health Statistics* (6). Series 14
   c. *Health, United States* (8). Under "Health Care Resources."
   d. American Medical Association publications (12).

7. *Financing*
   a. *Statistical Abstract of the United States* (1). Section 3.
   b. *Health, United States* (8). Under "Health Care Expenditures."
   c. *Guide to the Health Care Field* and *Hospital Statistics* (9). Certain financial data concerning hospitals.
   d. *Health Care Financing Review* (10).
   f. American Medical Association publications (12). Certain financial data concerning physicians.

Index

S

F
REC
I